实用医护英语
Practical Medical English

主 编 卢 芳 赵 琳 杨小蕾
副主编 杨 波 朱云萍 陈 波 胡 洋 万瑞雪

电子工业出版社·
Publishing House of Electronics Industry
北京·**BEIJING**

内 容 简 介

本书针对医学高等院校中成人教育部分设计，共分为八个主题鲜明的单元，每个单元围绕一个精心策划的主题，以卫生健康科普知识和真实医护情境及叙事展开。本书注重内容与其专业相结合、语言难易度适中，具有实用性与可操作性，力求贴近行业与实际工作场景，激发学习兴趣，强化语言实践能力。本教材也适用于对医疗健康话题感兴趣的英语爱好者。

图书在版编目（CIP）数据

实用医护英语 / 卢芳，赵琳，杨小蕾主编. -- 北京：
电子工业出版社，2024. 8. -- ISBN 978-7-121-48698-2

Ⅰ．R47

中国国家版本馆 CIP 数据核字第 2024QF6250 号

责任编辑：路　越
印　　刷：三河市良远印务有限公司
装　　订：三河市良远印务有限公司
出版发行：电子工业出版社
　　　　　北京市海淀区万寿路 173 信箱　　邮编：100036
开　　本：787×1092　1/16　印张：10.5　　字数：322 千字
版　　次：2024 年 8 月第 1 版
印　　次：2024 年 8 月第 1 次印刷
定　　价：56.80 元

本书编委会

主　编

　　卢　芳　赵　琳　杨小蕾

副 主 编

　　杨　波　朱云萍　陈　波　胡　洋　万瑞雪

参　编

　　吴　坚　杨克西　保林波　普璇华　范月红　孙静洋　陈　姗
　　潘梦妮　余　倩　王　巍　陶　然　张秀梅　秦金梅

前　言

在当今全球化的医疗环境中，英语作为国际交流的通用语言，在医疗卫生服务、专业信息获取和国际交流与合作中发挥着至关重要的作用。掌握好英语，无疑会为医护从业人员的职业发展打开更加广阔的大门。为了响应这一时代需求，并切实提高我国基层医疗机构医护人员的英语应用能力，我们特此精心编写了这本《实用医护英语》。

本书针对医学高等院校中成人教育部分设计，主要使用对象是医疗卫生行业的一线工作者。考虑到使用者群体的特点——明确的卫生医疗健康保健领域从业方向，拥有扎实的专业技能，但英语基础相对薄弱。本书特别注重内容与其专业相结合、语言难易度适中，具有实用性与可操作性，力求贴近行业与实际工作场景，激发学习兴趣，强化语言实践能力。

全书共分为八个主题鲜明的单元，每个单元围绕一个精心策划的主题，以卫生健康科普知识和真实医护情境及叙事展开，如公共卫生话题、常见病防治、未来医疗、医患故事等。本书既有卫生知识科普讲解，又涵盖国际医护领域的最新动态与新闻报道，还有记叙文形式展现的护理人员职业生活和感人故事，将语言、知识、情感、思政教育有机融为一体。通过课文学习，普及卫生健康知识，提升英语语言能力，培养仁爱医德。

在教学结构上，本书设置了"听与说"、"读与写"以及"语法聚焦"三大模块。"听与说"模块旨在通过医疗背景下的主题对话样板和对话练习提升读者在实际日常工作场景中应用英语进行口头沟通交流的能力；"读与写"模块通过精选的阅读材料，让读者熟悉常用的医学词汇与表达，培养读者用英语获取行业信息的阅读理解能力和书面表达自己观点的能力；而"语法聚焦"模块就常用的、读者容易使用不当的语法专项进行讲解和练习，帮助读者巩固语言、夯实基础，提升英语表达能力。

我们期望通过本书的学习，能够助力读者拓展国际视野，增强跨文化交际能力，从而更好地服务于日益多元化的患者群体，并在卫生行业的国际合作与交流中扮演更加积极的角色。同时，我们也鼓励读者将所学应用于日常工作，成为传播健康知识、促进社区福祉的有力使者。本书也适用于对医疗健康话题感兴趣的英语爱好者。

最后，感谢您选择这本教材，希望它成为您职场道路上的一座桥梁，连接起专业知识与英语语言，在英语学习和专业发展的道路上助您一臂之力，帮助您在面对医疗卫生事业国际化发展时更自信和从容。预祝您在此过程中取得丰硕的成果！

编者

2024 年 7 月

CONTENTS

Unit One　Medical Nursing

Listening & Speaking

Role-play

Listen to the following conversations, and play the role with your partner.

Dialogue One

Nurse: Good afternoon, madam. What can I do for you?

Patient: Good afternoon. Where is the registration office, please?

Nurse: Follow me, please. Look at that line over there. Those people are queuing for registration.

Patient: I have a stomachache. Which department should I register?

Nurse: You'd better go to the Digestive Department.

Patient: OK. Could you tell me how to get to the Digestive Department, please?

Nurse: Take the lift to the second floor. Turn left and you'll see the sign.

Patient: Thanks a lot.

Nurse: You are welcome.

Dialogue Two

Jack: Good morning, David. We haven't met for a while.

David: Morning, Jack. Yes, we haven't. You look tired. Are you OK?

Jack: I've been playing online games for months, and I feel great pain in my back and shoulders.

David: Sorry to hear that you're feeling under the weather. You should spend less time playing online games. Do you have any other hobbies?

Jack: Mm, I like watching movies in my spare time.

David: You should take some outdoor activities, such as swimming, mountain climbing and jogging.

Jack: But I am not interested in any of them.

David: How about playing football?

Jack: Oh, yes, I love it.

David: Well, we'll have a football match this Sunday afternoon at the football field of No.1 Middle School. Will you come and join us?

Jack: Sure, see you then!

David: See you!

Speaking Practice

Fill in each blank with the choice that best suits the situation until the dialogue is complete. Then play the role with your partner.

Dialogue One

Doctor: _____1_____

Mark: My head feels very hot and I feel a little dizzy.

Doctor: OK, let me take your temperature.

Mark: _____2_____

Doctor: Well, you have had a high fever.

Mark: _____3_____

Doctor: Don't worry. Just take this medicine three times a day and have a good rest, you'll be better soon.

Mark: Thank you.

A. Do I have a fever?

B. What seems to be the problem?

C. Do you feel better?

D. Is it serious?

Dialogue Two

Nurse: Good afternoon, Madam. How are you feeling today?

Sherry: I'm feeling much better._____4_____ The medicine is really effective.

Nurse: That's wonderful to hear! _____5_____

Sherry: Yes, I take one tablet twice a day.

Nurse: _____6_____

Sherry: No, not really. Should I be concerned?

Nurse: Yes, it will be better to lose some weight so that the pressure on your knees will be reduced a little.

Sherry: Alright. I'll make an effort to do that. Thank you.

Nurse: You are welcome.

A. Are you still taking Brufen?

B. Do you have any other hobbies?

C. Have you noticed any weight loss?

D. The pain has almost gone.

Dialogue Three

Nurse: Good afternoon, Mr. Johnson. I hope you're doing well. I wanted to inform you that your surgery is scheduled for tomorrow morning.

Mr.Johnson: Good afternoon, nurse. Thank you for informing me. What should I do before the surgery?

Nurse: _____7_____ as your surgery is set to begin at 8 AM tomorrow.

Mr. Johnson: I see. Is there any special requirement for the diet during the day?

Nurse: _____8_____ Mr. Johnson.

Mr. Johnson: Got it. Anything else should I be aware of?

Nurse: If you experience any discomfort or have any concerns before the operation, please let us know. Communication is crucial.

Mr. Johnson: OK. _____9_____

Nurse: You'd better rest in a supine position for the first 6 hours.

Mr. Johnson: I'll keep that in mind. Thank you so much!

Nurse: It's my pleasure. _____10_____

A. Do you have any advice for me after the surgery?

B. If you have any questions or concerns, please feel free to ask.

C. It's recommended to stick to a liquid diet today.

D. You should not take any food or liquid after 9 PM tonight.

Reading & Writing

Text A

The Essential Role of Nursing in Healthcare

In the realm of healthcare, nursing stands as a fundamental pillar, contributing significantly to the well-being of individuals and communities. This article explores the vital aspects of nursing, highlighting its pivotal role in patient care, education, and the ever-changing environment of modern healthcare.

Compassionate Patient Care: A Core Tenet of Nursing

The core of nursing revolves around the principle of providing compassionate care to patients, placing the patient's comfort and well-being at the forefront. Nurses <u>serve as</u> advocates, ensuring that individuals receive <u>personalized care</u> that not only addresses their physical health but also attends to their emotional and psychological needs. The empathy embedded in nursing practice profoundly impacts the overall patient experience.

Educating for Health and Preventive Care

Beyond hands-on patient care, nurses <u>play a crucial role</u> as educators and promoters of preventive health care. They empower individuals and communities with the knowledge and skills needed to <u>make informed decisions</u> about their health. Through health education initiatives, nurses significantly <u>contribute to</u> disease prevention and the promotion of healthy lifestyles, ultimately enhancing the overall health of populations.

Adapting to Technological Advances

Nurses are <u>at the forefront of</u> incorporating technological advancements into patient care. From electronic health records to advanced medical equipment, nurses adeptly navigate and utilize technology to improve the efficiency and quality of healthcare delivery. The ability to adapt to and embrace technological changes is a hallmark of modern nursing practice.

Collaborative Approach: Nursing in <u>Interprofessional Teams</u>

Nursing extends beyond individual care, involving collaboration within interprofessional healthcare teams. Nurses work seamlessly with physicians, therapists, and other healthcare professionals to ensure comprehensive and holistic patient care. This interdisciplinary approach facilitates effective communication and enhances healthcare outcomes, showcasing the interconnectedness of various healthcare disciplines.

Embracing Diversity in the Field of Nursing

Diversity is a cornerstone of nursing, not only within patient populations but also within the profession itself. Nurses come from various backgrounds, cultures, and experiences, contributing to the richness of healthcare. This diversity enables nurses to connect with patients on a personal level, fostering trust and understanding, particularly in multicultural and global healthcare settings.

Challenges and Opportunities in Nursing Education

Nursing education faces both challenges and opportunities in meeting the demands of a rapidly evolving healthcare landscape. The need for highly skilled and specialized nurses is <u>on the rise</u>. Nursing education programs must be adapted by incorporating innovative teaching methods, simulation technology, and ongoing professional development to prepare nurses for the complexities of modern healthcare.

　　In conclusion, nursing serves as a nurturing force in healthcare, encompassing compassion, education, technology, collaboration and diversity. As healthcare continues to evolve, the role of nurses becomes increasingly critical. Their unwavering dedication to patient well-being and their ability to adapt to the changing healthcare landscape make nursing an indispensable force in promoting health and healing in our communities.

(461 words)

New Words

healthcare [ˈhelθkeə]	**n.**卫生保健，医疗（保健）
realm [relm]	**n.**领域，范围；王国；（学术的）部门，界
fundamental [ˌfʌndəˈmentl]	**adj.**基础的；根深蒂固的；必需的；基音的
	n.原理
pillar [ˈpɪlə(r)]	**n.**柱，台柱，顶梁柱；墩，柱脚；（组织、制度、信仰等的）核心
highlight [ˈhaɪlaɪt]	**v.**突出，强调；（使）醒目；挑染
	n.最好的部分；挑染的头发；强光部分
pivotal [ˈpɪvətl]	**adj.** 关键的，中枢的；枢轴的
compassionate [kəmˈpæʃənət]	**adj.**有同情心的；表示同情的
tenet [ˈtenɪt]	**n.**原则；信条；教义
principle [ˈprɪnsəpl]	**n.**道德原则；法则；观念；理由；定律
advocate [ˈadvəkeɪt]	**vt.**拥护；主张；鼓吹
	n.拥护者，支持者；辩护律师
empathy [ˈempəθi]	**n.**<心>移情作用；同感，共鸣
embed [ɪmˈbed]	**v.**（使）嵌入；融入；派遣
preventive [prɪˈventɪv]	**adj.**预防的；防止的
empower [ɪmˈpaʊə(r)]	**vt.**授权；准许；使能够；使控制局势
initiative [ɪˈnɪʃətɪv]	**n.**主动性；主动精神；倡议；主动权
ultimately [ˈʌltɪmətli]	**adv.**最后，最终；基本上；根本

incorporate [ɪnˈkɔːpəreɪt]	vt.组成公司；包含；使混合；使具体化
	vi.包含；吸收；合并；混合
advancement [ədˈvɑːnsmənt]	n.发展，推动；提升，晋升
navigate [ˈnævɪgeɪt]	v.导航，确定路线；航行，航海；驾驭，
	成功应付（困难处境）
utilize [ˈjuːtəlaɪz]	vt.利用，使用
collaborative [kəˈlæbərətɪv]	adj.合作的，协作的
hallmark [ˈhɔːlmɑːk]	n.特点，标志；检验印记
	vt.给…盖上品质证明印记；使具有…标志
seamlessly [ˈsiːmləsli]	adv.无空隙地；无停顿地
holistic [həˈlɪstɪk]	adj.全盘的，整体的；功能整体性的
interdisciplinary [ˌɪntəˈdɪsəplɪnəri]	adj.各学科间的；跨学科
facilitate [fəˈsɪlɪteɪt]	v.促进；使便利
showcase [ˈʃəʊkeɪs]	v.展示（优点）
	n.（商店或博物馆等的）玻璃柜台，玻璃陈列柜
interconnectedness [ˌɪntə·kəˈnektnəs]	n.互联性
discipline [ˈdɪsəplɪn]	n.学科；训练；纪律；自制力；行为准则
diversity [daɪˈvɜːsəti]	n.多样性，多元性；差异，不同
cornerstone [ˈkɔːnəstəʊn]	n.基石，基础；最重要的部分
foster [ˈfɒstə(r)]	v.促进，鼓励，培养；代养，抚育
specialized [ˈspeʃəlaɪzd]	adj.专门的；专业的；专用的
innovative [ˈɪnəveɪtɪv]	adj.革新的；创新的；富有革新精神的
simulation [ˌsɪmjuˈleɪʃn]	n.模仿，模拟
complexity [kəmˈpleksəti]	n.复杂性
nurture [ˈnɜːtʃə(r)]	vt.养育；培育；滋养；培植
	n.教养，培育；营养物，食物；环境因素
encompass [ɪnˈkʌmpəs]	vt.围绕，包围；包含或包括某事物；完成
unwavering [ʌnˈweɪvərɪŋ]	adj.不动摇的，坚定的
indispensable [ˌɪndɪˈspensəbl]	adj.不可缺少的；绝对必要的；责无旁贷的；不可避开的

Phrases & Expressions

contribute to	促成；投稿；有助于
serve as	充当，担任；为

personalized care	个性化护理
play a crucial role	发挥关键作用
make informed decisions	做出明智的决定
adapt to	适应
at the forefront of	处于…最前列
interprofessional teams	跨专业团队
on the rise	在上涨[增长]；蓬勃高涨

Reading Comprehension

Choose the best answer to each of the following questions.

1. What is the core principle of nursing highlighted in the article? _____

A. Technological advancements

B. Compassionate patient care

C. Collaborative education

D. Administrative management

2. Apart from patient care, what role do nurses play in healthcare, according to the article?

_____

A. Administrative management

B. Advocates for preventive care

C. Primary focus on research

D. Limited involvement in health education

3. What is emphasized as a hallmark of modern nursing practice in the article? _____

A. Traditional patient care methods

B. Resistance to technological changes

C. Adaptation to and embrace of technology

D. Minimal interaction within healthcare teams

4. In the context of nursing, what does "interprofessional teams" refer to? _____

A. Individual patient care

B. Collaborative efforts within diverse teams

C. Nurse-led initiatives

D. Administrative tasks in healthcare

5. How does the article describe the role of diversity in nursing practice? _____

A. It is a challenge that needs to be overcome.

B. It is limited to patient populations.

C. It contributes to the richness of healthcare.

D. It creates barriers in patient communication.

Text B

A Nurse's Heartfelt Connection

Once upon a time in Sunflower Hospital, there was a kind-hearted nurse named Sarah. She had a special way of making patients feel cared for, and her days were filled with simple acts of kindness that <u>made a big difference</u>.

Sarah's journey into the nursing profession was not fueled by great ambitions, but by a genuine desire — to assist others. Her days were filled with a symphony of care, woven <u>together with</u> compassion, professional expertise, and a touch of kindness. The hospital corridors echoed with legends of Sarah's warm presence and the healing touch she brought to those who entrusted her with their care.

One of Sarah's patients, Mr. Brown, was an older gentleman with a friendly smile but a bit of loneliness in his eyes. He was admitted for some routine tests, but Sarah could sense that he needed more than just medical attention.

Sarah took a little extra time each day to sit and chat with Mr. Brown. She listened to his stories about his grandchildren, his love for gardening, and the adventures of his youth. In the midst of beeping machines, their conversations turned the hospital room into a place of warmth and companionship.

To brighten up Mr. Brown's space, Sarah brought in a small potted plant and placed it by the window. The room that once felt cold now had a touch of nature and cheer. She even played some soft music in the background, turning the hospital room into a more comforting environment.

Sarah's caring nature didn't <u>go unnoticed</u>. Mr. Brown's family, grateful for the extra attention, could see that their loved one was not just another patient but someone receiving personalized and compassionate care.

One evening, as the sun set, Sarah noticed a hint of sadness in Mr. Brown's eyes. Sensing that he might be feeling alone, she offered to stay a bit longer. Sarah rearranged her schedule to spend more time with him, providing the comfort and company he needed during the evening hours.

As the days passed, Mr. Brown's health improved not only because of the medical care but also because of the genuine care and attention he received from Sarah. The small gestures, like the potted plant and the extra time spent talking, <u>made a big impact on</u> his well-being.

Sarah's story became a source of inspiration in Sunflower Hospital. It wasn't about complicated medical procedures, it was about recognizing the person behind the patient and offering kindness in simple ways.

Her approach to nursing spread positive vibes throughout the hospital, reminding everyone that a friendly smile, a listening ear, and a bit of extra care could make a hospital stay more than just a medical experience — it could become a time of healing for the heart and soul. And so, in Sunflower Hospital, the story of Sarah, the nurse with a heart full of compassion, continued to brighten the days of those she cared for.

（485 words）

New Words

profession [prəˈfeʃn]	n.职业；业内人士；全体人员
ambition [æmˈbɪʃn]	n.追求，理想；雄心，野心
symphony [ˈsɪmfəni]	n.交响乐，交响曲
expertise [ˌekspɜːˈtiːz]	n 专门技术，专门知识；专长
echo [ˈekəʊ]	v.回响；发出回声；重复，附和
	n.回声；重复，附和；再现
entrust [ɪnˈtrʌst]	v.委托，托付
companionship [kəmˈpæniənʃɪp]	n.友谊；伴侣关系
grateful [ˈɡreɪtfl]	adj.感激的；表示感谢的
hint [hɪnt]	n 线索，迹象；提示，注意事项；暗示
	v.暗示
rearrange [ˌriːəˈreɪndʒ]	vt.重新安排；重新布置；改变既定的（计划等）
inspiration [ˌɪnspəˈreɪʃn]	n.灵感；鼓舞人心/启发灵感的人或事
procedure [prəˈsiːdʒə(r)]	n.程序，手续；工序，过程，步骤
spread [spred]	v.开展；伸开；传播；涂；分摊
	n.散布；广泛；酱；范围
vibe [vaɪb]	n.感应；气氛
brighten [ˈbraɪtn]	v.照亮，使更艳丽；露出喜色；（眼睛）发亮；（使）变得乐观；放晴

Phrases & Expressions

make a big difference	产生很大的不同；意义重大；有很大影响

together with	和…—起
go unnoticed	未被察觉的，不被注意到的
make a big impact on	对…产生重大影响

Reading Comprehension

Choose the best answer to each of the following questions.

1. Who is the main character in the story? _____

A. Mrs. Thompson

B. Mr. Brown

C. Lily

D. Sarah

2. What extra efforts does Sarah make to create a comforting environment for the patient? _____

A. Bringing in a small potted plant and playing soft music

B. Administering extra medications

C. Strictly adhering to hospital policies

D. Ignoring the patient's stories

3. Why did Mr. Brown's family appreciate Sarah's care? _____

A. She only focused on medical procedures.

B. She rearranged the hospital schedule.

C. She avoided personal conversations.

D. She provided personalized and compassionate care.

4. What transformation occurs in the hospital room due to Sarah's actions? _____

A. It becomes colder and more clinical.

B. It turns into a place of warmth and companionship.

C. It remains unchanged.

D. It becomes noisy and uncomfortable.

5. What is the primary message conveyed by the article about the role of the nurse, Sarah, in patient care? _____

A. Strict adherence to hospital policies is crucial.

B. Medical procedures are the sole focus of nursing.

C. Simple acts of kindness and compassion enhance patient well-being.

D. Nurses should avoid personal connections with patients.

Language Practice

I. Vocabulary and Structure

Directions: *Choose the one that best completes the sentence.*

1. The English Speaking Competition _____ the best in her. As a result, she is more active now.

A. checked out　　B. tried out　　　　C. brought out　　　　D. left out

2. When father saw my face, he knew _____ that something was wrong.

A. similarly　　B. immediately　　C. frequently　　　　D. fortunately

3. The leaders realize that a new crisis has _____ .

A. risen　　　　B. raised　　　　C. regarded　　　　D. arisen

4. You'd better leave now, _____ you'll miss the last train.

A. if else　　　B. as well　　　　C. or else　　　　D. or not

5. _____ you were coming today, I'd have met you at the bus station.

A. Had I known　B. Have I known　　C. I had known　　D. I have known

6. If I had the time, I _____ on a holiday like that in France.

A. will go　　　B. had gone　　　C. would have gone　D. would go

7. If you were the manager of human resources department, what would you do _____ the current situation?

A. improving　　B. having improved　C. to improve　　　D. to have improved

8. During the last two decades, the number of people participating in physical fitness programs _____ sharply.

A. were decreased　B. have decreased　　C. has decreased　　D. had decreased

9. Tracy's poor English has _____ misunderstanding between her and her American boss.

A. resulted in　　B. resulted from　　C. due to　　　　D. come from

10. The Chinese language has become a bridge to _____ China _____ the rest of the world.

A. translate; into　B. connect; to　　C. separate; from　　D. compare; with

11. A lot of museums in China are worth _____. If you have time, you can have a visit.

A. to visit　　　B. visit　　　　C. visited　　　　D. visiting

12. I have some tickets for the basketball match. I called my friends to see _____.

A. when did we go together　　　　B. whether they'd like to go

C. where did they buy them   D. why they liked to go there

13. _____, a naughty child has many wild and crazy thoughts.

A. In person   B. In public   C. In case   D. In general

14. David will give us a report as soon as he _____.

A. arrived   B. will arrive   C. arrives   D. is arriving

15. Hardly _____ the room when the telephone rang.

A. I got to   B. had I got to   C. did I get to   D. I had got to

16. Mrs. Green was good at making _____ flowers from cloth, which looked so real.

A. artificial   B. artistic   C. artist   D. article

17. Animals may not be as _____ as humans, but they are smart in different ways.

A. intelligence   B. intelligent   C. more intelligent   D. more intelligence

18. Lucy was busy doing homework _____ Tom was playing basketball.

A. unless   B. until   C. while   D. whether

19. _____ trying and do your best!

A. To keep   B. Keeping   C. Keep   D. Kept

20. Finding out these museums has become easy for anyone with Internet _____.

A. entrance   B. entry   C. admission   D. access

II. Cloze

Directions：*Choose the best one to complete the passage.*

Hospitals are the places for the medical treatment and care of individuals who are ill or sick, or in need of medical attention, for example, in pregnancy. Additionally, they can function as hubs for medical research and serve as educational institutions for training doctors, nurses, and other _____1_____ workers.

Hospitals can be categorized as general or specialized. The general hospitals have many different _____2_____ like medical, surgical, obstetric, pediatric, dental, gynecological and traditional medicine department. People of all ages, with different illnesses and injuries, can receive treatment at general hospitals. Conversely, specialized hospitals _____3_____ particular areas of care. _____4_____, some specialize in treating patients with chronic conditions, providing facilities for long-term care, while others take patients of only one age group, such as children, or patients with one particular illness, such as mental disorder.

A hospital mainly _____5_____ two major departments: the out-patient department and the in-patient department. Additionally, there is an emergency room. There are consulting rooms in the out-patient department. And there are wards and intensive care units in the in-patient department. Wards can be classified into several types, such as medical, surgical, maternity, isolation, and observation wards, each equipped with hospital beds.

Doctors, nurses and other medical workers make up the ___6___ of a hospital. Doctors are specialized in various fields such as physicians, surgeons, dentists, eye-doctors and ear-nose-throat doctors. Both doctors and nurses provide care for the patients. However, for doctors, the primary ___7___ is on the science of medicine. It is often said that doctors focus on treating diseases while nurses focus on caring for patients. ___8___ patients often have short daily interactions with their doctors. ___9___, they have more frequent encounters with nurses, as nurses are ___10___ for the majority of patient care in hospitals and are present around the clock, monitoring patients continuously.

1. A. physical   B. medical   C. educational   D. scientific

2. A. departments   B. offices   C. buildings   D. colleges

3. A. keep on   B. depend on   C. focus on   D. insist on

4. A. For one thing   B. For sure   C. For instance   D. For ages

5. A. composes of   B. separates   C. divides into   D. consists of

6. A. staff   B. leader   C. official   D. entrepreneur

7. A. method   B. measure   C. strategy   D. emphasis

8. A. Unhappy   B. Depressed   C. Hospitalized   D. Sick

9. A. In a hurry   B. In contrast   C. In a word   D. In time

10. A. useful   B. competent   C. respectable   D. responsible

III. Translation

Directions: *Translate the following passage into Chinese.*

Communication skills are important in everyday life, but in the medical field, these skills can be the difference between life and death. Active listening skills are critical for effective patient-centered care, especially for obtaining important medical information. Active listening shows patients that you care and establishes a foundation of trust. Body language is just as important as what you say during a conversation. Maintain eye contact and nod at appropriate times to show you are actively engaged in what your patient has to say. Avoiding crossing your arms and keeping an open posture to show you are open to communication. Avoiding grimaces and frowns, which can discourage patients from sharing personal information due to embarrassment.

be critical for	对…至关重要
be engaged in	从事（于）

grimace ['grɪməs]	**n.** 做鬼脸，怪相
frown [fraʊn]	**n.** 皱眉；不同意
discourage sb. from doing sth.	阻止，阻拦，劝阻
embarrassment [ɪmˈbærəsmənt]	**n.** 尴尬；难堪（的事）

IV. Writing

Directions: *You are to write on the topic "**What Attitude Should I Take to Money**". You should base your composition on the Chinese outline given below and your essay should not be less than 100 words.*

1. 社会上人们对金钱的错误看法。

2. 分析批驳这种错误的观点。

3. 提出自己的观点。

Grammar Focus

★复合句

根据从句引导功能不同，复合句大致可以分为：宾语从句、定语从句、状语从句等。

一、宾语从句

宾语从句是一种名词性从句，在句子中作及物动词的宾语、介词的宾语。

1. 宾语从句的时态

（1）主句是一般现在时，从句根据需要选用相应的时态。

例如：<u>Do</u> you <u>know</u> when the meet <u>will begin</u>?

（2）主句的谓语是一般过去时，从句的谓语动词在时态上要用相应的过去时态。

例如：I <u>wondered</u> why Laura <u>was</u> absent from school yesterday.

（3）若从句表示的是客观真理或自然现象，无论主句是什么时态，从句都用一般现在时态。

例如：Scientists <u>have proved</u> that the earth <u>rotates</u> around the sun.

2. 宾语从句的语序

宾语从句的语序应为陈述句的语序。

例如：Do you know which class <u>he is</u> in?

　　　Can you tell me how <u>I can get</u> to the train station?

3. 宾语从句的分类：

根据引导宾语从句的不同连词，宾语从句可以分为三类。

（1）由 if 或 whether 引导的宾语从句，if 和 whether 在句中的意思为"是否"。

例如：Mark asked me whether/if I could wait for him.

　　　 I want to know if/whether she lives there.

（2）由 that 引导的宾语从句。that 没有实在意义，仅起到语法作用，在非正式表达中可以省略。

例如：My boss hopes (that) everything goes well.

　　　 I believe (that) she can achieve success.

（3）由连接代词 which、who、whom、whose、what 和连接副词 where、when、why、how 等引导的宾语从句。

例如：Please go and find out when the bus will arrive.

　　　 These songs express exactly what people feel about love, life and relationships.

二、定语从句

定语从句在句中作定语，用来修饰某一个名词、名词词组或者代词。被定语从句修饰的词称为先行词，引导定语从句的关联词有关系代词和关系副词。

1. 关系代词

关系代词有 which、that、who、whom、whose。

（1）which 指物，在从句中作主语或宾语，作宾语时在非正式语体中可以省略。

例如：The museum (which) we visited last week is located in the suburb of Kunming.

（2）that 多指物，有时也可以用来指人，在从句中作主语或宾语。

例如：The room that once felt cold now had a touch of nature and cheer.

　　　 Who is the man that is playing basketball?

（3）who 指人，在从句中作主语。

例如：The girl who is wearing a hat is clever.

（4）whom 指人，在从句中作宾语，有时可以省略。

例如：Do you know the young woman (whom) we met at the airport?

（5）whose 指人或物，在从句中只能用作定语。

例如：Please pass me the book whose cover is blue.

2. 关系副词

关系副词有 when、where、 why。如果要修饰方式，用 that 或 in which 引导，或者不用引导词。

（1）when 指时间，在从句中作状语。

例如：I will never forget the day when we were in Dali.

（2）where 指地点，在从句中作状语。

例如：The museum where her mother works is in the south of the city.

（3）why 指原因，在从句中作状语。

例如：Is it the reason why she refused our offer?

3. 具体使用时需要注意以下几点。

（1）只能用 which，不用 that 的情况

在非限制性定语从句中通常用 which 作引导词，而不能用 that 作非限制性定语从句的引导词。

例如：The trees, which were planted by my friend five years ago, have grown up.

定语从句由"介词+ 关系代词"引导，先行词是物时，

例如：They are all questions to which there are no answers.

（2）只能用 that，不用 which 的情况

先行词为 all、everything、anything、nothing、little 等不定代词时，

例如：All (that) she lacked was training.

先行词是形容词最高级或被形容词最高级修饰的词时，

例如：This is the best film that I have ever seen this year.

先行词被序数词和 the last 修饰时，

例如：Jason was the first one that told me the secret.

先行词中既有人又有物时，

例如：They talked about the engineers and the factories that they had visited.

主句是含有 who 或 which 的特殊疑问句，为了避免重复时，

例如：Who is the woman that you spoke to just now?

三、状语从句

用来修饰主句中的动词、形容词和副词或整个句子的从句称为状语从句。状语从句主要分为时间状语从句、地点状语从句、原因状语从句、条件状语从句、目的状语从句、结果状语从句、让步状语从句、方式状语从句。

1. 时间状语从句

时间状语从句常用 when、while、as、since、until、till、as soon as、before、after

等词来引导。需要注意的是，如果主句是一般将来时，从句只能用一般现在时表示将来意义。

例如：I will ring you up as soon as I get to Beijing.

She had learned a little English before she came to London.

2. 地点状语从句

地点状语从句通常由 where 引导。

例如：Where there is a will, there is a way.

3. 原因状语从句

原因状语从句常用 because、since 和 as 引导，但需要注意其差别。because 语气最强，用来说明人们所不知道的原因，回答 why 提出的问题。当原因是显而易见的或已为人们所知的，就用 as 或 since。

例如：Tom didn't go, because he was afraid.

As it is raining, we shall not go to the park.

4. 条件状语从句

条件状语从句常用 if、unless、as long as、on condition that 等词引导，谓语动词通常用现在时态表示将来的动作或状态。

例如：Where shall we go if it rains tomorrow?

I will not go to the supermarket unless I am free tomorrow.

5. 目的状语从句

目的状语从句由 that、so that、in order that、in case 等词引导。

例如：You must speak louder in order that you can be heard by all.

6. 结果状语从句

结果状语从句常由 so…that、such…that 引导。so 是副词，只能修饰形容词或副词，such 是形容词，修饰名词或名词词组。

例如：The girl is so young that she can't go to school.

She is such a young girl that she can't go to school.

7. 让步状语从句

让步状语从句常由 although、though 等词引导。需要注意的是，当有 though、although 时，后面的从句不能有 but，但是 though 和 yet 可以连用。

例如：Although I was exhausted, I had to go on working.

Though she is living alone, she is very happy.

8. 方式状语从句

方式状语从句通常由 as、(just) as…so…、as if、as though 引导。需要注意的是，as if 和 as though 两者的意义和用法相同，引出的状语从句谓语多用虚拟语气，表示与事实相反，有时也用陈述语气，表示所说情况是事实或实现的可能性较大。

例如：When in Rome, do <u>as</u> the Romans do.

I completely ignore these facts <u>as if (as though)</u> they never existed.

Have a check on your grammar 过关演练

Directions: *Choose the best answer to complete the sentence.*

1. I plan to go to the Yunnan Museum, but I'm not sure _____.

A. how can I get there   B. how I can get there

C. how am I there   D. how I am there

2. If she _____ a three-week holiday next year, I will take part in a short study tour to Zhejiang University.

A. takes   B. took   C. will take   D. is taking

3. Yesterday Li Jiao went to the farm _____ her family lived five years ago.

A. where   B. which   C. when   D. that

4. _____ it's really difficult to make his dream come true, he never gives up.

A. Because   B. If   C. Unless   D. Though

5. They are talking about the piano and the pianist _____ were in the concert last week.

A. whom   B. who   C. that   D. which

Unit Two　Doctor–patient Communication

Listening & Speaking

Role-play

Listen to the following conversations, and play the role with your partner.

Dialogue One

Doctor: What brings you in today?

Patient: I have a fever.

Doctor: Alright, that's a common issue. Can you tell me how long you've been experiencing the fever?

Patient: I'm not exactly sure. I think it started yesterday.

Doctor: Okay, have you taken any medications to try to bring it down?

Patient: No, I haven't.

Doctor: Well, there's a good chance that you might have a viral infection, possibly a cold or flu, given the fever. Since it's relatively high, I want to rule out infection first.

Patient: I understand.

Doctor: Let's discuss your options. I'll prescribe you some over-the-counter medication called acetaminophen. It's very effective at reducing fevers, and I think it's safe to take for at least three days.

Patient: I'm okay with taking it for three days.

Doctor: You might have some minor side effects from taking it, but they are usually manageable.

Patient: Okay, sounds good.

Doctor: I'll write you a prescription for a two-day supply to ensure your recovery.

Patient: I understand.

Doctor: I'd like you to come back in one week to make sure you're feeling better. If you're still unwell, we might consider a different prescription.

Patient: That sounds good.

Doctor: I'll see you next week.

Patient: Thank you, Doctor.

Dialogue Two

(*The family member visits the doctor again with new reports in hand.*)

Doctor: The cancer is at a stage just before spreading to other parts. In this case, the best course of action is quick surgery to remove the affected area, followed by radiation therapy.

Family member: How long will the treatment take?

Doctor: We can perform the operation in a couple of days. Consequently, we will monitor the patient for 4-5 days. Radiation therapy is well-regulated now, and your father can get it done in any tier-2 city, which not only benefits you but also reduces costs.

Family member: I understand, and what about the duration of the radiation therapy? How long will it take my father to complete it?

Doctor: Your father will need one dose every two weeks for three months. He only has to visit the hospital on therapy days. After completing radiation, regular consultations with an oncologist are necessary every three months initially and then annually to check for cancer cell remission.

Family member: OK. I've heard radiation therapy has side effects. What will the side effects be in my father's case?

Doctor: Yes, there are potential side effects, including hair loss, loss of appetite, and nausea, the feeling of impending vomiting.

Family member: I see. Thank you, doctor. We will get him admitted today.

Speaking Practice

Fill in each blank with the choice that best suits the situation until the dialogue is complete. Then play the role with your partner.

Dialogue One

Patient: Good morning, I need to schedule an appointment to see a doctor.

Nurse: Good morning! ___1___ Could you please tell me your name and the reason for your visit?

Patient: Hi, my name is Alice Johnson, and I've been experiencing severe back pain in the past week. I think I might need to see a specialist.

Nurse: ___2___ Ms. Johnson. We do have such a specialist available, Dr. Brown. Let me check his schedule.

[Checking the system]

Nurse: Alright, Alice. Dr. Brown has an opening next Wednesday at 2 PM. ___3___

Patient: That's quite soon, actually. Yes, that works for me. Can you please book that slot for me?

Nurse: Of course, I'm scheduling you in for an appointment with Dr.Brown on Wednesday, March 1st at 2 PM. Please make sure to arrive 15 minutes early to complete any necessary preparations. Also, remember to bring your ID, insurance card, and a list of any medications you're currently taking.

Patient: Great, thank you very much. Will there be any special preparations required before the appointment?

Nurse: It would be helpful if you could avoid eating or drinking anything other than water for about two hours prior to your appointment as some tests may require fasting. If there are specific instructions from Dr. Brown's office, we will send them via email or text message to you.

Patient: Understand. I'll make sure to follow those instructions. Thanks again.

Nurse: You're welcome, Alice. If you have to change or cancel your appointment, please give us a call at least 24 hours in advance. Have a good day and take care until then!

Patient: I will. Thanks. See you on Wednesday.

Nurse: Looking forward to it, Ms. Johnson. Take care, and we'll see you next week.

A. You're welcome.

B. What can I assist you today?

C. Would that work for you?

D. Thank you for letting me know,

Dialogue Two

Patient: Hello, I'm here for my scheduled appointment with Dr. Brown at 2 PM.

Nurse: Good afternoon, Madam. Welcome to our clinic. My name is Nurse Sophia. Before we move forward, ___4___

Patient: Sure, it's Alice Johnson, and my date of birth is May 15th, 1980.

Nurse: Thank you, Mrs. Johnson. Yes, I see your appointment right here. Have you filled out the new patient forms or updated your information since your last visit?

Patient: Yes, I've completed them online earlier today.

Nurse: Great. ___5___ Perfect, everything looks up-to-date. Now, how are you feeling today? Are you experiencing any discomfort or new symptoms?

Patient: Actually, I've been experiencing severe back pain in the past week. That's why I came in today.

Nurse: I see. We'll definitely make sure the doctor is aware of this. Please take a seat and I will inform Dr. Smith of your arrival. Your blood pressure and weight will be taken shortly as well.___6___

Patient: No, that covers the main concerns. But I do have a question about medication refills.

Nurse: Of course, feel free to tell me about it, and we can discuss it with Dr. Brown during your consultation.

Patient: Alright, thank you. It's regarding my prescription for hypertension.

Nurse: Understood, I'll make a note of that. The doctor will be with you shortly, Mrs. Johnson. If you need anything in the meantime, just let me or any of our staff know.

Patient: Thank you very much, Nurse Sophia.

Nurse: You're welcome, Mrs. Johnson. Have a seat, and we'll call you in when we're ready.

A. I will check if Dr. Brown is available now.

B. Let me just double-check that they've come through on our system.

C. May I have your full name and the date of birth for verification?

D. Is there anything else you'd like to mention before I let the doctor know?

Dialogue Three

Nurse: Good morning, Mrs. Johnson. I'm Nurse Sarah.___7___

Alice Johnson: Hi, Nurse Sarah. To be honest, my back pain has been quite unbearable overnight. It's really distressing me and making it difficult for me to move or even turn over in bed.

Nurse Sarah:___8___Alice. Let me check your chart to see if there have been any updates from the doctor regarding your condition. Have you taken your prescribed pain medication as directed?

Alice Johnson: Yes, I took the last dose around 7 AM, but unfortunately, the relief wasn't substantial. The pain seems to persist and intensify when I try to sit up or shift positions.

Nurse Sarah: I understand.___9___In the meantime, would you like me to arrange a warm compress for your back or perhaps ask for an additional dose of pain relief medication if it's due?

Alice Johnson: A warm compress sounds helpful. And yes, please discuss with the doctor if it's possible to increase or change my medication to manage this pain better.

Nurse Sarah: Absolutely, Alice. We'll get that arranged right away. Also, ___10___

Alice Johnson: It's a deep, throbbing ache mainly centralized in my lower back area, and it doesn't seem to spread to my legs. But every time I cough or sneeze, it feels like a knife stabbing me.

Nurse Sarah: Thank you for that detailed description, Alice. That will help the medical team evaluate your case more accurately. I'll also inquire about scheduling a physical therapy session or a consultation with a specialist during doctors' rounds if needed. We want to ensure we're addressing all aspects of your discomfort.

Alice Johnson: That would be appreciated, Nurse Sarah.

Nurse Sarah: You're welcome, Alice. Rest assured that we're here to provide you with the best possible care. If your pain worsens or if you need anything at all, please don't hesitate to press your call button. I'll check back on you soon.

Alice Johnson: Thank you very much for your assistance, Nurse Sarah.

A. How are you feeling today?

B. Could you describe the nature of the pain? Is it localized, sharp, dull, or does it radiate anywhere else?

C. I'll inform your attending physician about the lack of improvement with your current pain management plan.

D. I'm sorry to hear that,

Reading & Writing

Text A

Window Treatment

Candice, a young woman who had been enduring extremely painful skin problems since the age of 14, was finally diagnosed with hidradenitis suppurativa at the prestigious Johns Hopkins Hospital when she turned 17. Over the years, her life revolved around many episodes of sore outbreaks, surgeries to treat them, and lots of emotional pain. She had to go through skin grafts, muscle flaps, and plenty of tears — it felt like an endless loop.

Having spent 12,456 days in hospital, Candice stopped counting after realizing that most of her life had been spent as a patient. She said, "I've missed out on so much, looking out windows that don't let me into the world outside."

Our team met Candice during one of her stays at Johns Hopkins Bayview for treatments related to her condition. During those initial weeks, she expressed her frustration with the unsuccessful attempts to heal her. While gazing out the window, she would often wonder who she truly was, feeling lost because of all the physical changes she'd endured.

Candice found strength from remembering her mother, who stood by her side through every challenge until she passed away when Candice was 23. Her mother's resilience lived on within her.

Enter Felicia, who was affectionately called "my light" by Candice. Felicia was her nurse for several months, observing Candice's loneliness and boredom during her extended hospital stay. To help, she asked Candice about her sources of happiness, and Candice mentioned that creating art brought her joy.

Felicia then came up with a brilliant idea. One morning, she surprised Candice with washable window markers and suggested they make a mural together. At first, Candice thought drawing on the window was a bit odd and left the markers untouched for about one month, fearing she might damage the glass. However, they eventually decided to give it a try. Felicia drew a small, easily removable smiley face and heart in the corner to prove it wouldn't be permanent.

One day, after a tough therapy session, Candice picked up the markers and started drawing in the middle pane of the window. Her nurse that day joined in, sketching her dream pet — a pug and a bird eating a worm. And just like that, the project took off! Everyone who visited Candice's room, including doctors, nurses, and cleaning staff, added their own drawings to the window. They created animals, nature scenes, and messages filled with encouragement.

For example, Candice invited David, her palliative care doctor, to add his artwork to the collection. He quickly drew Snoopy and Woodstock, sharing a story from his childhood when he drew something similar for his second-grade teacher. His teacher proudly displayed the drawing, which reminded him of the power of art to bring people closer together.

Day after day, the window transformed into a colorful collage, eventually covering all three panes. The leaders of the unit also supported the initiative and contributed their own drawings. Candice felt immense happiness seeing others participate, making the original concept of a single planned mural unnecessary. The collective artwork, crafted organically by dozens of healthcare team members, turned out to be far more inspiring than any meticulously designed piece could have been. It showed that the combined creativity and support of many can create something truly magical and uplifting.

(549 words)

New Words

endure [ɪnˈdjʊə(r)]	**v.**忍受；持续
diagnosis [ˌdaɪəgˈnəʊsɪs]	**n.**诊断；判断
hidradenitis [hɪdræˈdenaɪtɪs]	**n.** [医] 汗腺炎
suppurativa	**adj.** 化脓性的
prestigious [preˈstɪdʒəs]	**adj.** 受尊敬的，有声望的
revolve [rɪˈvɒlv]	**v.**（使）旋转，环绕，转动；围绕
episode [ˈepɪsəʊd]	**n.**一集，一节；插曲，一段经历；（病症）发作期
sore [sɔː(r)]	**adj.**疼痛的；使人伤心的；恼火的，发怒的
	n.（肌肤的）痛处，伤处
outbreak [ˈaʊtbreɪk]	**n.**（战争，怒气等的）爆发；突然发生
surgery [ˈsɜːdʒəri]	**n.**外科学，外科手术；手术室；诊所；诊断时间
emotional [ɪˈməʊʃənl]	**adj.**感情的；有感染力的；情绪激动的
graft [grɑːft]	**n.**移植；嫁接；渎职；贪污，受贿
	vt.移植；嫁接；接枝；贪污；用嫁接法种植
	vi.移植；贪污；受贿；嫁接
muscle [ˈmʌsl]	**n.** 肌肉；力量；权威，权力
flap [flæp]	**v.**振（翅）；摆动，挥动；拍打
	n.拍打；扁平下垂物；襟翼；激动，忧虑
muscle flaps	肌肉皮瓣
loop [luːp]	**n.**圈，环；[医]宫内避孕环；回路；弯曲部分
	v.（使）成环，（使）成圈；以环连结；使翻筋斗
initial [ɪˈnɪʃl]	**adj.**开始的
	n.首字母
	v.用姓名的首字母签名于
frustration [frʌˈstreɪʃn]	**n.**挫折；失败；挫败；失意
attempt [əˈtempt]	**v.**努力，尝试，企图
	n.努力，尝试，（杀人）企图
heal [hiːl]	**v.**（使）康复；治愈；（使）结束
challenge [ˈtʃælɪndʒ]	**n.**挑战；比赛邀请；质疑
	v.对…怀疑；挑战，考验；盘问

resilience [rɪˈzɪliəns]	**n.**弹性；弹力；快速恢复的能力；回弹
affectionately [əˈfekʃənətlɪ]	**adv.**挚爱地，亲切地；脉；脉脉
boredom [ˈbɔːdəm]	**n.**讨厌，令人讨厌的事物；无聊，无趣；厌倦
extend [ɪkˈstend]	**v.**延长；扩展，扩大；提供
brilliant [ˈbrɪliənt]	**adj.**巧妙的；使人印象深的；聪颖的；技艺高超的；非常好的；成功的；鲜明的；明亮的；灿烂的
mural [ˈmjʊərəl]	**n.**（通常指大型的）壁画
smiley [ˈsmaɪli]	**n.**笑容符，用：-）表示
permanent [ˈpɜːmənənt]	**adj.**永久的；不断出现的；终生的；固定的
	n.卷发
therapy [ˈθerəpi]	**n.**治疗，疗法，疗效；心理治疗；治疗力
session [ˈseʃn]	**n.**会议；开庭；一段时间；学年
	adj.伴奏的
pane [peɪn]	**n.**窗玻璃；窗格；嵌板；方框
sketch [sketʃ]	**n.**草图；素描；梗概
	v.草拟；速写；简述
pug [pʌg]	**n.**哈巴狗；泥料；拳师；（兽）脚印
scene [siːn]	**n.**地点，现场；场面；镜头；圈子，坛；景色；风景画；争吵
message [ˈmesɪdʒ]	**n.**音信；信息；电邮；要旨；购物
	v.给…发消息
palliative [ˈpæliətɪv]	**n.**治标药物；缓解剂；治标措施；保守疗法
collage [ˈkɒlɑːʒ]	**n.**拼贴画；大杂烩；拼贴艺术
initiative [ɪˈnɪʃətɪv]	**n.**主动性；主动精神；倡议；主动权
contribute [kənˈtrɪbjuːt]	**v.**捐献；增加，增进；做贡献；促成；撰稿；讲话；是…的原因
craft [krɑːft]	**n.**手艺，技巧，手腕；船；飞行器
	v.精心制作
organically [ɔːˈgænɪklɪ]	**adv.**器官上地，有机地；逐渐的；演进的；自然的
inspire [ɪnˈspaɪə(r)]	**v.**激励；启发；赋予灵感；唤起（感情）；吸入（空气）
meticulously [məˈtɪkjələslɪ]	**adv.**过细地，异常细致地；无微不至；精心
combine [kənˈbaɪn , ˈkɒmbaɪn]	**v.**使结合，混合；融合；协力，联合；同时做；（人）兼具，兼有；（使）结合；（使）联合；（使）合并；（使）综合
	n.联盟，集团；联合收割机

uplift [ˈʌplɪft]	**vt.**举起；振作；（社会、道德等）发展；使上升
	vi.上升，升起

Phrases & Expressions

revolve around	围绕…旋转/绕转；环绕，以…为中心
go through	经历；度过；通读
feel like	摸起来像是…，有…的感觉；想要…
miss out on	错过；错失
relate to	与…相关；涉及；谈到
feel lost	怅然若失；恍然若失；不知所措
pass away	去世
come up with	想出，想到
surprise sb. with sth.	用…使（某人）惊奇
give it a try	试一试
pick up	拿起；提起；捡起；取走；学会；（身体）恢复，好转
take off	脱掉；起飞；（使）离开；突然成功
fill with	（使）充[挤]满；使满怀（某种情感等）
remind sb. of sth.	提醒某人某事
transform into	把…转变成…
turn out to be	结果是，原来是，证明是

Reading Comprehension

Choose the best answer to each of the following questions.

1. What diagnosis did Candice receive at the age of 17? _____

   A. Eczema   B. Psoriasis

   C. Hidradenitis Suppurativa   D. Acne Vulgaris

2. How long had Candice spent in hospitals by the time she stopped counting her days there? _____

   A. Approximately 3 years and 9 months   B. Approximately 34 years

   C. Approximately 14 years   D. Approximately 17 years

3. Who gave Candice washable window markers to create art together during her hospital stay? _____

   A. Her mother   B. David, her palliative care doctor

C. Felicia, her nurse   D. The leader of the unit

4. What inspired Candice's nurse to suggest making a mural on the window? _____

A. Candice's boredom and love for art

B. A childhood memory of Candice's

C. An initiative from the hospital's arts program

D. A suggestion from Candice's therapist

5. Why was the collaborative artwork created on Candice's window so special?_____

A. It was designed by a famous artist.

B. It symbolized the resilience of one individual overcoming adversity.

C. It was later sold to raise funds for medical research.

D. It brought together various healthcare professionals and visitors, creating a sense of community and support.

Text B

Just Relax and Concentrate on Your Breathing

When someone with asthma experiences a severe attack and goes to the <u>emergency room</u>, they often hear the advice, "Just try to calm down and <u>focus on</u> your breathing." This suggestion is meant to be soothing, but for many patients in the middle of an asthma flare-up, it can actually create more anxiety. As an individual living with severe asthma who has faced this situation multiple times, I know that during an attack, focusing too much on my breath can be scary because I'm struggling to breathe normally and might worry about what could happen if things don't improve.

During these tough moments, even though speaking is difficult, many people with asthma, including me, still make an effort to communicate. Talking helps us <u>shift</u> our attention <u>away</u> from the fear of not being able to breathe by giving us something else to <u>concentrate on</u>. It might look like a big effort, but talking can actually help ease the panic and <u>prevent</u> us <u>from</u> <u>getting caught up</u> in a cycle where we over-focus on our breathing and accidentally hyperventilate.

When I first arrive at the ER(Emergency Room) during an asthma attack, the medical staff's top priority is to understand my situation. For individuals with <u>long-term</u> or difficult-to-control asthma, we usually have lots of knowledge about what treatments work best for us personally. At times, I've noticed doctors discussing treatment options without asking me directly. Despite the considerable effort required to communicate, having someone take the time to listen provides <u>a huge sense of</u> comfort, almost as helpful as taking medicine like IV magnesium or aminophylline. Knowing that the doctors have the important information needed for my treatment makes me feel safer.

To make it easier when talking is tough, healthcare workers can give patients a pen and paper to write down their thoughts. By including patients in decisions about their care, even if it means writing <u>instead of</u> talking, they feel more involved and confident <u>in their care process</u>.

Individuals respond to asthma attacks in various ways. In my case, sitting upright or leaning forward feels more comfortable than lying back. Instead of consistently advising patients to lie down and relax, which can be overwhelming for some, it's better for the medical team to ask patients to find a position that works best for them. This simple adjustment can <u>make a</u> big <u>difference</u> in how comfortable and cooperative a patient is during their examination and treatment.

I am fortunate that my local hospital now uses a special plan for people with ongoing health issues or complex needs. Once I <u>get admitted to</u> the ER, the staff can quickly access my personalized anticipatory care plan. Since they started using this, my visits to the emergency department have been much better. The doctors and nurses immediately have the necessary information about my asthma history and usual treatments, eliminating the pressure for me to explain everything <u>right away</u>. This understanding lets me relax, knowing that I'll receive the right treatment tailored to my specific needs, <u>rather than</u> worrying that they might use a treatment that could make my asthma worse.

（523 words）

New Words

asthma [ˈæsmə]	**n.** <医>气喘，哮喘
emergency [iˈmɜːdʒənsi]	**n.**紧急事件
	adj.紧急情况下的；应急的
soothe [suːð]	**vt.**安慰；缓和；使平静；减轻痛苦
flare-up [ˈfleərˌʌp]	**n.**火焰、光等的骤发或骤燃；激怒；怒气（或疾病）的发作；昙花一现式的出名
multiple [ˈmʌltɪpl]	**adj.**多重的；多个的；复杂的；多功能的
	n.<数>倍数；[电工学]并联；连锁商店；下有多个分社的旅行社
scary [ˈskeəri]	**adj.**使人惊慌的；胆小的，容易受惊的；可怕的，吓人的
communicate [kəˈmjuːnɪkeɪt]	**v.**沟通；传递；传染；相通

attention [əˈtenʃn]	n.注意（力）；兴趣，关注；照料，维修；殷勤
	int. 注意！立正！
concentrate [ˈkɒnsntreɪt]	v.全神贯注；使集中；使浓缩
	n.浓缩液；
panic [ˈpænɪk]	n.恐慌；恐慌局面
	v.使惊慌失措
hyperventilate [ˌhaɪpəˈventɪleɪt]	[医]过度呼吸
priority [praɪˈɒrəti]	n.优先，优先权；重点
option [ˈɒpʃn]	n.选择；选择权；可选择的事物
comfort [ˈkʌmfət]	n.舒适；安逸生活；安慰；感到安慰的人/物；使生活舒适的东西
	v.安慰
magnesium [mægˈni:ziəm]	n.[化]镁（金属元素）
aminophylline [ˈæmɪnɒfɪlaɪn]	n.氨茶碱
involve [ɪnˈvɒlv]	v.包含，涉及；（使）加入；表明…
confident [ˈkɒnfɪdənt]	adj.坚信的；自信的；肯定的
upright [ˈʌpraɪt]	adj.直立的；正直的；规矩的
	n.立柱
overwhelm [ˌəʊvəˈwelm]	v.使不知所措，使难以承受；淹没；征服，压倒，击败（感情或感觉）充溢
adjustment [əˈdʒʌstmənt]	n.调整，调节； 转变
ongoing [ˈɒnɡəʊɪŋ]	adj.不间断的，进行的；前进的
issue [ˈɪʃu:]	n.问题；（报刊）期号；发行；子嗣
	v.发表，发布；供给；出版；将…诉诸法律
complex [ˈkɒmpleks]	adj.复杂的；复合的
	n.综合建筑群；相关联的一组事物；复合体；情结；忧虑
access [ˈækses]	n.入口，通道；（使用或见到的）机会/权利
	v.访问，存取（计算机信息）；到达，进入，使用
anticipatory [ænˌtɪsɪˈpeɪtəri]	adj.期待着的；提早发生的
tailor [ˈteɪlə(r)]	n.裁缝
	v.专门制作；订做

Phrases & Expressions

| emergency room | <美>急诊室 |

focus on	集中；特别关注
shift away	搬走
concentrate on	集中精力于
prevent from	阻止，防止
get caught up	被卷入，卷入到
long-term	长期的；近期难以有所改变/解决的
a sense of	一种…感觉
instead of	（用…）代替…，（是…）而不是…，（用…）而不用…
in the process	在此过程中（表示一种未想到或不希望的情况）
make a difference	有作用或影响
get admitted to	被录取
right away	立刻，马上；就；当时
rather than	而不是

Reading Comprehension

Choose the best answer to each of the following questions.

1. What common advice do patients with asthma often receive during severe attacks in the emergency room, and why can it be counterproductive? _____

    A. Take deep breaths; because it might lead to hyperventilation

    B. Focus on your breathing; because it could increase anxiety

    C. Stay calm and don't talk; because it conserves energy

    D. Lie down and relax; because it improves lung function

2. Why do some people with asthma still try to communicate during an attack despite the difficulty? _____

    A. To distract themselves from the fear of not being able to breathe

    B. To provide medical history to the healthcare workers quickly

    C. To demonstrate their ability to control the situation

    D. To prevent over-medication by doctors

3. What does the author suggest is a better approach for healthcare workers when advising patients on their position during an asthma attack? _____

    A. Always advise patients to lie down

    B. Encourage patients to stand up and relax

    C. Ask patients to find a position that works best for them

    D. Consistently advise patients to lie down and relax

4. According to the passage, what is a more inclusive approach for healthcare workers to take when communicating with patients who find talking difficult during an asthma attack? _____

A. Asking patients to write down their symptoms and preferences

B. Speaking louder and slower to help them understand

C. Encouraging patients to lie down and rest until they can speak

D. Deciding on treatments based on general guidelines

5. How has the anticipatory care plan at the author's local hospital improved their experience in the emergency department? _____

A. By providing immediate relief through personalized medicine

B. By reducing wait times and expediting treatment

C. By giving medical staff access to the patient's specific health information and treatments

D. By allowing patients to bring a support person to assist with communication

Language Practice

I. Vocabulary and Structure

Directions: *Choose the one that best completes the sentence.*

1. The athlete experienced intense _____ when he was disqualified despite being on track for a gold medal finish.

A. joy   B. anxiety   C. frustration   D. relief

2. To explain his new invention, the engineer made a rough _____ on a piece of paper to visualize its design.

A. drawing   B. sketch   C. model   D. diagram

3. Tattoos are considered a _____ form of body art because they last for the lifetime of the individual.

A. temporary   B. changeable   C. permanent   D. occasional

4. After moving to a new city without knowing anyone, Jane initially _____ and struggled to find her way around.

A. felt lost   B. found comfort   C. made friends easily   D. got settled quickly

5. Over the course of several weeks, the caterpillar _____ a beautiful butterfly.

A. became into   B. divided into   C. adapted as   D. transformed into

6. During an asthma attack, patients are often advised to stay _____ in order to manage their symptoms more effectively.

A. tense   B. relaxed   C. anxious   D. agitated

7. The hospital has set up a dedicated _____ department to handle unexpected medical crises and urgent health issues around the clock.

A. outpatient   B. intensive care   C. emergency   D. surgical

8. During an asthma attack, it can be challenging to _____ effectively due to shortness of breath and anxiety.

A. communicate   B. collaborate   C. contemplate   D. celebrate

9. In modern healthcare, there has been a notable trend towards _____ from traditional hospital-centered models to more patient-centered care.

A. shifting away   B. moving forward

C. stepping aside   D. turning around

10. In her memoirs, the author wrote that during her early years as a painter, she _____ developing her skills in watercolor techniques.

A. centered around   B. focused in

C. immersed herself by   D. concentrated on

11. The _____ of the group are highly skilled professionals with years of experience.

A. members   B. participants   C. individuals   D. associates

12. The boss asked _____ to complete the project as soon as possible.

A. they   B. them   C. their   D. theirs

13. The _____ car was the most expensive model in the showroom.

A. late   B. later   C. latter   D. latest

14. The children ran _____ down the hill, laughing and shouting.

A. gaily   B. noisily   C. quickly   D. excitedly

15. We _____the project by the end of next month.

A. complete   B. will complete

C. will have completed   D. have completed

16. The homework _____ before class starts.

A. must finish   B. must be finished C. can finish   D. can be finishing

17. She enjoys _____ in the morning, which helps her to start the day with energy.

A. walking   B. to walk   C. walk   D. walked

18. The reason why he was late for class was _____ he overslept this morning.

A. because   B. that   C. due to   D. for

19. Either you or one of your colleagues _____ responsible for the delay.

A. are   B. were   C. is   D. be

20. The group _____ in the laboratory all night, trying to solve the problem.

A. worked   B. have worked   C. had worked   D. were working

II. Cloze

Directions: *Choose the best one to complete the passage.*

In June 2018, a 50-year-old lady who had recently been diagnosed with rheumatoid arthritis（类风湿性关节炎）visited the Emergency Department at Patan Hospital. She ___1___ repeated vomiting and painful mouth sores for five days straight. Her joint pain troubles began about one year ago, ___2___ led her to seek medical help in New Delhi where her son lived. There, she was told she had RA and ___3___ common medicines: 15 mg of methotrexate（甲氨蝶呤）once every week and 5 mg of folic acid（叶酸）two times each week. However, there was a mix-up -- she misunderstood and ___4___ 15 mg of methotrexate daily for 11 days instead.

After these 11 days, feeling very unwell, she went to National Medical College and Teaching Hospital near her home in Birgunj, Nepal. The doctors there discovered that she had several sore spots inside her mouth and tests showed her blood counts were low, indicating too ___5___ methotrexate. As a result, she was sent to our hospital for special care.

When she arrived, we stopped the methotrexate ___6___ and started her on different treatments: leucovorin （亚叶酸, a daily dose of 15 mg）, GM-CSF（粒-巨噬细胞集落刺激因子, 300 μg daily）, and feeding through a tube because her mouth sores made eating too painful. After staying in the Intensive Care Unit（ICU）for three days to make sure she was stable, she was moved to a ___7___ hospital room to continue these treatments.

She stayed in the hospital ___8___ everything improved – this took 11 days. By then, her blood cells, hemoglobin（血色素）, and platelets（血小板）returned to healthy levels, and her mouth sores healed enough for her to eat normally again. We restarted her on the correct dose of methotrexate (15 mg once a week) and spent extra time ___9___ her condition, how to take her medicines the right way, and what potential side effects might happen. Since then, she has been coming back to the rheumatology（风湿病学）clinic every three months. Now she is successfully managing her RA and is now taking her medications as instructed.

This story shows how important it is to communicate clearly and educate patients well. If the healthcare providers ___10___ that methotrexate should be taken weekly, this problem could have been prevented altogether.

1. A. experienced　　　　　　　　　B. has experienced
　 C. had experienced　　　　　　　　D. had been experiencing
2. A. it　　　　　B. that　　　　　C. which　　　　　D. when
3. A. prescribed　　B. described　　C. written　　　　D. ordered
4. A. ate　　　　　B. took　　　　　C. gave　　　　　D. has
5. A. many　　　　B. much　　　　　C. lot　　　　　　D. amount

6. A. rightly 　　B. at right 　　C. right away 　　D. immediate

7. A. regular 　　B. usual 　　C. plain 　　D. public

8. A. when 　　B. after 　　C. unless 　　D. until

9. A. explain 　　B. to explain 　　C. explaining 　　D. explained

10. A. emphasize 　　B. had emphasized 　　C. have emphasized 　　D. were emphasizing

III. Translation

Directions: *Translate the following passage into Chinese.*

In the world of healthcare, talking to and understanding each other is super important. When doctors talk to their patients really well, it can make a big difference in how happy and healthy people feel. A research study from 2008 found out that when doctors and patients have trouble communicating, it can cause more problems that could have been avoided, especially with medicines. It is reported that about 27% of mistakes made by doctors happen because they didn't communicate well.

When doctors and patients talk clearly, it helps avoid mistakes and keeps patients safer. But when communication isn't good, it can lead to bad things like patients not following their treatment plans, feeling unhappy with their care, or using medical resources in a wasteful way.

In South Asia, the usual way doctors are taught doesn't put much focus on learning how to talk to patients effectively. They mainly learn about the technical parts of being a doctor. Improving how doctors are taught to communicate could help them take better care of their patients and make sure everyone gets the best possible health results.

take care of 照顾；处理

IV. Writing

Directions: *You are to write on the topic "**Communication between doctors and patients**". You should base your composition on the Chinese outline given below and your essay should not be less than 100 words.*

1. 医患沟通的重要性。

2. 当前医患沟通的现状。

3. 如何改进医患沟通。

Grammar Focus

★主谓一致

英语中的主谓一致是指英语句子中谓语动词要与主语保持一致。它遵守语法一致、意义一致和就近原则三个原则。

一、语法一致

指英语句子中谓语动词与主语在单复数形式上保持一致。具体而言，主语是单数形式，谓语也用单数形式；主语是复数形式，谓语也用复数形式。

例如：The son enjoys playing computer games.

The parents enjoy watching TV.

以下是容易用错的几种情况。

1. 不定代词（either、neither、somebody、everybody、anybody、something、everything、anything、nobody、nothing、each 等）作主语，或修饰主语时，主语应视为单数，对应的谓语动词用单数：

例如：Everything seems perfect.

Somebody is knocking at the door.

Every boy and girl has the right to get good education.

Many a man has tried and failed in that endeavor.（形式上是单数，意义上表达的是复数，即许多人尝试却失败了。）

2. 不定式、动名词或者从句作主语，主语视为单数，谓语动词用单数。

例如：To learn a foreign language is challenging.

(= It is challenging to learn a foreign language. 不定式作主语时，往往用 it 作形式主语置于句首代替主语，将真正的不定式主语置于句尾，避免句子头重脚轻。)

Cooking at home can save money and is healthier compared to eating out.

What he said surprised everyone present.

二、意义一致

英语句子中，谓语动词的单复数形式要根据主语表达的意义来决定，无论主语以单数或者复数形式出现，当它表达的意义是单数时，谓语用单数；当它表达的意义是复数时，谓语用复数。

例如：My family is the most important thing in my life.（我的家庭，视为一个整体，谓语用单数）

My family are all gathering for the Spring Festival. （我们全家人，指家庭成员，谓语用复数）

以下几种情况容易出错。

1. 表示国家、机构、事件、作品、学科等词语作主语时，尽管主语词汇的形式是复数或者以-s 结尾，但是表达的是一个概念，视为单数，谓语动词用单数。

例如：The United Nations plays an important role in the international affairs.

Statistics is difficult to learn.

New York Times has a wide circulation.

2. 主语后面有 as well as、as much as、accompanied by、including、in addition to、more than、no less than、rather than、together with 等引导的短语，该短语不影响主语的单复数，它们其实是状语，在句中的位置可以变化，谓语动词应该跳过它们与主语保持一致。

例如：The manager, together with his colleagues, is working tirelessly to meet the project deadline.

（=Together with his colleagues, the manager is working tirelessly to meet the project deadline.

= The manager is working tirelessly to meet the project deadline, together with his colleagues.）

3. and 连接两个主语时，如果在意义上是指同一人、物、事或者概念时，谓语用单数，指两种不同的人、物、事或者概念时，谓语用复数。

例如：War and Peace is a constant theme in history.

Rice and wheat are both staple foods.

4. 一个单数名词作主语，同时被两个不同的形容词修饰，如果表示的是不同的概念，谓语用复数，如果表示的是相同的概念，谓语用单数。

例如：White and black coffee sell well here.

(=White coffee and black coffee sell well here.)

The large and spacious house is what many people dream of.

5. 表示时间、距离、金额、重量、计量、空间、体积等意义的复数名词作主语时，可以看成一个整体，谓语动词用单数。

例如：Eight hours of sleep is enough.

Four from twenty-four leaves twenty.

三、就近原则

英语句子中，当用 or、either…or、neither…nor、not only…but also…等连词连接并列主语时，谓语动词的人称和数与最接近它的主语词语保持一致，这就是就近原则。

例如：Either you or I am responsible for it.

Either I or you are responsible for it.

在由 here、there、where 等引导的倒装句中，谓语动词也遵守就近原则。

例如：Here is a pen and some pieces of paper for you.

Have a check on your grammar 过关演练

Directions: *Choose the best answer to complete the sentence.*

1. A series of lectures on artificial intelligence _____ for next month, attracting many enthusiasts in the field.

    A. has scheduled   B. is scheduled

    C. have scheduled   D. are scheduled

2. The team, including its coach, _____ determined to win the championship this year.

    A. is   B. are   C. has   D. have

3. Mathematics _____ my favorite subject in high school.

    A. is   B. are   C. be   D. were

4. Neither John nor his friends _____ seen the new movie yet.

    A. is   B. are   C. has   D. have

5. Bread and butter _____ for a satisfying breakfast in many countries.

    A. make   B. makes   C. is made   D. are made

Unit Three   Influenza

Listening & Speaking

Role-play

Listen to the following conversations, and play the role with your partner.

Dialogue One

Doctor: Good morning. What's troubling you?

Patient: Good morning, doctor. I am experiencing a terrible headache.

Doctor: I see. Could you tell me how it started?

Patient: Yesterday, I had a runny nose. Now it is stuffed up and my throat is sore. I think I might have got a fever. I'm feeling unwell.

Doctor: There is no need to worry, young man. Let's have an examination. First, I will check your throat. Please open your mouth and say "ah".

Patient: Ah.

Doctor: Good. Now extend your tongue out. All right, let me examine your chest next. Please unbutton your shirt so that I can check your heart and lungs. Take a deep breath and hold it. Breathe in deeply, and then out. By the way, do you have a history of tuberculosis?

Patient: No, definitely not.

Doctor: Look, your throat appears inflamed and your tongue is thickly coated. It seems that you're suffering from influenza.

Patient: What should I do then, doctor?

Doctor: All you need is plenty of rest. I'll write you a prescription.

Patient: Thank you very much, doctor.

Doctor: You're welcome. Make sure to take a good rest and drink more water.

Patient: I will, doctor. Goodbye.

Doctor: Bye!

Dialogue Two

Rose: Tim, you don't look well today. Are you okay?

Tim: I think I might have caught a cold. I keep coughing and feel aches all over.

Rose: Sounds a bit like the flu. A common symptom of the flu is body aches. Remember, Mike and Pam both came down with the flu last week and are on sick leave now.

Tim: Hmmm, maybe you're right. I do feel like I'm running a fever, too.

Rose: You should consider taking a sick day. See a doctor and get some medicine.

Tim: You are right. I will do that.

Rose: Take good care of yourself. Hope you get well soon.

Tim: Thanks! Bye.

Speaking Practice

Fill in each blank with the choice that best suits the situation until the dialogue is complete. Then play the role with your partner.

Dialogue One

A: _____1_____

B: Yes, I've been down with a cold for the past few days and it's really uncomfortable

A: That doesn't sound pleasant. _____2_____

B: Not yet. I don't think it's a big problem, so I've just been resting at home and drinking hot water, but there's been no significant improvement in my condition.

A: Maybe you should consult with a doctor or, at least, get some over-the-counter cold medicine

B: Yeah, I plan to see a doctor tomorrow. _____3_____

A: Definitely! Drink more hot water, stick to light meals, and ensure plenty of rest. And importantly, always wear a mask to prevent spreading it to others around you.

B: Alright, thanks for these suggestions. I hope I'll get better soon.

A. Have you seen a doctor?

B. What seems to be the problem?

C. Have you caught a cold recently?

D. Do you have any recommendations for me?

Dialogue Two

Nurse: Good afternoon, Madam. How are you feeling today?

Sherry: I'm feeling much better._____4_____ The medicine is really effective.

Nurse: That's wonderful to hear! _____5_____

Sherry: Yes, I take one tablet twice a day.

Nurse: _____6_____

Sherry: No, not really. Should I be concerned?

Nurse: Yes, it will be better to lose some weight so that the pressure on your knees will be reduced a little.

Sherry: Alright. I'll make an effort to do that. Thank you.

Nurse: You are welcome.

A. Are you still taking Brufen?

B. Do you have any other hobbies?

C. Have you noticed any weight loss?

D. The pain has almost gone.

Dialogue Three

A: Hello, Daniel speaking, what may I help you?

B: Hi, Daniel, it's Julie.

A: Hi, Julie, how are you doing today?

B: Actually. _____7_____

A: Oh, no, that's concerning. What's wrong?

B: It looks like I've caught the flu. I have a headache, a sore throat, a runny nose and

_____8_____

A: I'm sorry to hear that. _____9_____

B: Yes, I was hoping to take a day off to recover.

A: Alright then. Make sure _____10_____ and take care of yourself.

A. I'm feeling slightly feverish.

B. I'm feeling quite ill today.

C. you get plenty of rest.

D. So you're calling in sick for today?

Reading & Writing

Text A

Reflections on Pandemics: Past, Present, and the Path Forward

Although more than six months have already passed after the World Health Organization declared COVID-19 a pandemic, people still puzzle over an unanswered question: How will it ultimately come to an end?

It seems reasonable to assume that someday, in some way, it will indeed come to an end. After all, other viral pandemics have. For example, the flu pandemic of 1918–1919 was the deadliest in the 20th century, infecting about 500 million people and killing at least 50 million worldwide, with 675,000 individuals in the U.S alone. Even though science has made significantly advancements since then, the uncertainty experienced globally today would have been familiar a century ago. In fact, even after that virus died out, scientists took years to gain a better understanding about what had happened. Up to now, certain mysteries still remain.

What we understand so far is that a pandemic will not come to an end until the disease in question has reached a point where it is unable to successfully find enough hosts to catch and spread it. In the case of the 1918 flu, it swept the world in 1918 and 1919, but cases spiked again in early 1920. According to Howard Markel, a physician and director of the Center for the History of Medicine at the University of Michigan, flu strains may have become more active in the winter because people were spending more time indoors in closer proximity to one another, and viruses can enter skin cracks caused by artificial heat and fires.

It wasn't until the middle of 1920 that the pandemic was finally subsided in many regions, without any official declaration. "The end of the pandemic occurred because the virus circulated around the globe, infecting enough people that the world population no longer had enough susceptible people for the strain to become a pandemic again," explains J. Alexander Navarro, a medical historian and Markel's colleague, who serves as the assistant director of the Center for the History of Medicine.

Eventually, with "fewer susceptible people out and about and mingling," Navarro says, there was nowhere for the virus to go. This is what we now call "herd immunity". By the time it faded out, a whopping one-third of the world's population had caught the virus. Today, about half a percent of the global population has been infected with novel coronavirus.

However, the end of the 1918 pandemic wasn't just the result of so many people catching it. Social distancing was also key factor to reducing its impact. Public-health guidelines back then were strikingly similar to today's recommendations. People were urged to wear masks and wash hands frequently. Patients were quarantined and isolated, and schools and public spaces were closed.

A study published in the Journal of the American Medical Association in 2007 found that U.S. cities that implemented more than one of these control measures earlier and maintained them longer experienced less severe and deadly outcomes than those that implemented fewer measures later. Public-health officials took these measures even though they were not sure whether they were dealing with a virus or a bacterial infection; it wasn't until the 1930s that the research proved influenza comes from a virus, and the articles published in Science and Nature in 2005 capped off the process of mapping the genome of the 1918 strain.

Currently, scientists are still learning the behavior of COVID-19, but they expect the pandemic won't really end before both a vaccine becomes available and a certain level of exposure is achieved in the global population. In the meantime, the public can make an effort to limit the impact of the pandemic. A century ago, proactive public health measures saved lives, and they can certainly do so again in the present day.

(620 words)

New Words

pandemic [pænˈdemɪk]	adj.（疾病）大规模流行的
	n. <正式>大流行病
viral [ˈvaɪrəl]	adj.病毒的；病毒性的；病毒引起的
infect [ɪnˈfekt]	v.传染；使感染；影响
host [həʊst]	n.主人，东道主；节目主持人；宿主
	v.主办，主持
spike [spaɪk]	n.猛增，急升；尖状物；尖头；尖刺
	v.用尖物刺入（或扎破）
strain [streɪn]	n.压力；拉力；张力；品种，类型
	v.损伤；拉伤；扭伤 尽力；竭力；使劲
proximity [prɑːkˈsɪməti]	n.（时间或空间）接近，邻近，靠近
artificial [ˌɑːtɪˈfɪʃ(ə)l]	adj.人造的，人工的；人为的
declaration [ˌdekləˈreɪʃn]	n.声明，表白；公告，宣告
circulate [ˈsɜːkjəleɪt]	v.（液体或气体）环流，循环，传播；流传；散布
susceptible [səˈseptəbl]	adj.易受影响（或伤害等）；敏感；过敏
mingle [ˈmɪŋɡl]	v.（使）与…结合；使混合；使联结
whopping [ˈwɒpɪŋ]	adj.巨大的；很大的
novel coronavirus	新型冠状病毒
impact [ˈɪmpækt , ɪmˈpækt]	n.巨大影响；强大作用 撞击；冲撞；冲击力
	v.（对某事物）有影响，有作用；冲击；撞击
quarantine [ˈkwɒrəntiːn]	n.（为防传染的）隔离期；检疫
isolate [ˈaɪsəleɪt]	v.孤立，分离；隔离
implement [ˈɪmplɪmənt]	v.使生效；贯彻；执行；实施

influenza [ˌɪnfluˈenzə]	**n.**同 flu，流行性感冒；流感
bacterium [bækˈtɪriəm]	**n.**细菌；bacteria 的单数
exposure [ɪkˈspoʊʒər]	**n.**暴露，接触；曝光，揭发

Phrases & Expressions

come to an end	结束，完结，告终
die out	消失，灭绝，逐渐消失，熄灭
in question	被提及的；讨论中的；相关的
herd immunity	群体免疫
be similar to	类似于，与什么一样
know for sure	确切知道
cap off	完成，结束
in the meantime	在此期间，同时

Reading Comprehension

Choose the best answer to each of the following questions.

1. When did the flu pandemic of 1918–1919 end? _____

A. In early 1920

B. In the middle of 1920

C. After World War I

D. After World War II

2. What was a key factor in reducing the impact of the 1918 pandemic? _____

A. Social distancing

B. Quarantine only

C. Masking only

D. Frequent hand washing only

3. What did public-health advice during the 1918 pandemic urge people to do? _____

A. Go out more often

B. Wear masks and wash hands frequently

C. Open schools and public spaces

D. Refuse to wash hands

4. According to the article, what percentage of the global population is known to have been infected with the novel coronavirus? _____

A. About 5%

B. About 10%

C. About 50%

D. About 0.5%

5. What do scientists expect will happen before the COVID-19 pandemic really ends?

_____

A. There will be a vaccine for the common cold.

B. There will be a certain level of exposure in the global population.

C. There will be a cure for cancer.

D. There will be world peace.

Text B

Follow These 3 Steps to Fight the Flu

Influenza，commonly known as the flu, is a contagious disease that can be severe. Almost every year, the flu causes illness in millions of persons, with hundreds of thousands getting hospitalized and tens of thousands dying. The health authorities such as the Centers for Disease Control and Prevention (CDC), urge you to take the following measures to protect yourself and others from the flu.

1. Get vaccinated

The first and most important step to protect you against flu viruses is to get a flu vaccine each year. Ideally, everyone older than 6 months should receive a flu vaccine before the end of October, or as soon as possible afterward.

Flu vaccines are available in many places, such as physician offices, clinics, health departments, drugstores, and university health centers, and sometimes through employers or schools.

Getting vaccinated can not only reduce your risk of getting sick with flu but also make your condition less severe in case you do catch it. Even if you have had the flu within the season, this vaccine can still protect you from getting sick with other influenza viruses that may be spreading. Vaccination may also help protect vulnerable people around you, such as infants, young children, older people, pregnant women, and people with certain chronic health conditions. Annual flu vaccination for everyone above 6 months old is the best protection against the flu.

Therefore, get vaccinated to protect yourself and your family.

2. Avoid contact

To prevent infection, you should avoid any close contact with sick people, refrain from touching your eyes, nose, and mouth. When coughing or sneezing, cover your nose and mouth with a paper towel, and throw it into the garbage bin after using it. Remember to wash your hands frequently with soap and water, and clean and sanitize surfaces and objects that may be contaminated with flu viruses.

If you get sick, minimize your contact with other people as much as possible. Stay at home until at least 24 hours after the fever is gone, except to receive necessary medical care. Make sure that your fever has disappeared for about 24 hours without using a drug to decrease it before resuming your regular activities.

3. Take antiviral drugs if prescribed by your doctor

If you catch the flu, antiviral drugs can be used to treat it.

Antiviral drugs can alleviate the symptoms, shorten the duration of the disease, and prevent serious complications like pneumonia.

The CDC recommends the use of antiviral drugs during the early stages of treatment for patients who are severely affected by the flu, particularly those hospitalized or at high risk of severe complications due to their age or underlying health conditions.

(453 words)

New Words

contagious [kənˈteɪdʒəs]	**adj.**（病）接触传染的；（态度）感染性的
severe [sɪˈvɪə(r)]	**adj.**十分严重的，极为恶劣的；艰巨的，严峻的
hospitalize [ˈhɒspɪtəlaɪz]	**vt.**住院；入院就医
urge [ɜːdʒ]	**v.**敦促，催促，力劝；竭力主张，强烈要求；驱赶，鞭策；鼓励
	n.强烈的欲望，冲动；推动力
measure [ˈmeʒə(r)]	**n.**措施，办法；适量，适度；判断，衡量
vaccinate [ˈvæksɪneɪt]	**v.**给…接种疫苗；接种疫苗
offer [ˈɔːfər]	**v.**提供，给予；提议；出（价）；提出
physician [fɪˈzɪʃ(ə)n]	**n.**医师，（尤指）内科医生
clinic [ˈklɪnɪk]	**n.**诊所，门诊部；门诊时间；（医院的）科，室
drugstore [ˈdrʌgstɔːr]	**n.** [药] 药房（常兼售化妆品、杂志等杂货）
avoid [əˈvɔɪd]	**v.** 避免，防止；回避，避开
cough [kɒf]	**v.** 咳嗽；（从喉咙或肺中）咳出
	n. 咳嗽（病）；咳嗽声
sneeze [sniːz]	**v.** 打喷嚏

	n. 打喷嚏，喷嚏声
contaminate　[kənˈtæməneɪt]	adj.受污染的，被感染的, 弄脏的
	v.污染；玷污，毒害
decrease [dɪˈkriːs]	v.（使）减少，（使）降低
	n.减少，降低
resume [rɪˈzjuːm]	v.（中断后）重新开始，继续
regular [ˈregjələr]	adj.定期的，规律的；经常的，频繁的；惯常的，通常的
alleviate [əˈliːvieɪt]	v.减轻，缓和
prevent [prɪˈvent]	v.阻止，阻碍；防止，预防
recommend [ˌrekəˈmend]	v.建议，劝告；推荐，介绍

Phrases & Expressions

in millions of	数百万，以百万计
hundreds of thousands	数以十万计的，成千上万的
take measures to	采取措施
protect yourself against flu viruses	保护自己免受流感病毒的侵害
garbage bin	垃圾箱或垃圾桶
except to	除了，不包括
catch the flu	感冒，患流感
due to	由于，因为

Reading Comprehension

Choose the best answer to each of the following questions.

1. Who should get a flu vaccine each year? _____

A. Only children under 6 months of age

B. Only adults over 60 years old

C. All persons 6 months of age or older

D. Only pregnant women

2. Why should you and your family get vaccinated against the flu? _____

A. To prevent a common cold

B. To protect yourself and others from the flu viruses

C. To avoid contact with sick people

D. To reduce the risk of hospitalization and death

3. When should you get a flu vaccine each year? _____

A. Before the end of October

B. After October

C. Anytime during the year

D. Only if you feel sick

4. Where can you get a flu vaccine? _____

A. Only at physician offices

B. Only at drugstores

C. At many places, such as physician offices, clinics, health departments, drugstores, and university health centers, as well as from many employers and even at some schools

D. Only at hospitals

5. What can antiviral drugs do for someone who catches the flu? _____

A. Alleviate the symptoms

B. Shorten the duration of the disease

C. Prevent serious complications

D. All of the above

Language Practice

I. Vocabulary and Structure

Directions: *Choose the one that best completes the sentence.*

1. "Influenza" is a _____ disease.

A. contagious   B. non-contagious   C. temporary   D. genetic

2. The _____ is the main way to prevent influenza.

A. antiviral   B. vaccine   C. mask   D. sanitizer

3. If a person has symptoms of the flu, it means they are infected with the _____.

A. virus   B. bacteria   C. antibodies   D. vaccines

4. The new product had a significant _____ on the market, selling over a million units in its first month.

A. effect   B. result   C. impact   D. consequence

5. Prolonged _____ to sunlight can cause skin damage and increase the risk of skin cancer.

A. contact   B. exposure   C. affection   D. exposition

6. You can't hear what I'm saying _____ you stop talking.

A. only if   B. unless   C. lest   D. except that

7. He _____ working till he was seventy years old.

A. kept up   B. kept on   C. kept to   D. kept out

8. The novel ended happily, and the young couple was married _____.

A. in the final   B. in the end   C. to the last   D. in conclusion

9. One warning was _____ to stop her doing it.

A. suffered   B. sufficed   C. suggested   D. provided

10. It is estimated that the disease _____ by polluted water will kill 1 out of every 100 children.

A. causing   B. caused   C. to cause   D. will cause

11. He didn't know I was in his office. He was too busy to _____ me.

A. pay attention to   B. notice   C. know   D. realize

12. Will you show me the girl _____ name is Jane?

A. her   B. who' s   C. whose   D. which

13. Mr. Holmes called at many schools _____ he lived to ask them to accept his son, but he was refused everywhere for being a black.

A. that   B. around where   C. near which   D. which

14. My wallet is nowhere to be found. I _____ when I was on the bus.

A. must drop it   B. should have dropped it

C. must have dropped it   D. had dropped it

15. I could have done it better if I _____ more time.

A. have had   B. had   C. had had   D. will have had

16. _____, we should be glad.

A. They arrive tomorrow   B. Were they arriving tomorrow

B. They were to arrive tomorrow   D. Were they to arrive tomorrow

17. I knew I could not finish my homework _____.

A. by him had come   B. until he came

C. when he comes   D. before he comes

18. It is not _____ that this situation will last very long.

A. alike   B. the like   C. like   D. likely

19. I _____ on seeing the manager. The service in this hotel is terrible.

A. insist   B. persist   C. affirm   D. protest

20. Experienced teachers make _____ mistakes than beginners.

A. lesser   B. fewer   C. not many   D. very few

II. Cloze

Directions: *Choose the best one to complete the passage.*

Social distancing measures, _____1_____ to slow the spread of COVID-19, may have an unexpected benefit: reducing the spread of other diseases. NBC News'Medical Correspondent Dr. John Torres believes these measures could be _____2_____ the spread of other infectious diseases, including the flu.

Torres points to Australia as an example. "During the winter months, when the flu is usually _____3_____, early figures show influenza rates are at a record low this year," he said. "Hospitals are seeing _____4_____ cases compared to previous years."

Other countries are also reporting _____5_____ trends. Canada and the UK have reported exceptionally low levels of influenza, while China, where lockdown measures were first widely enforced, has seen a decline in mumps and measles cases. Torres believes these results are not _____6_____ and attribute them to the widespread use of preventative measures like masking, hand washing, and social distancing.

"Like COVID-19, flu, measles, and mumps are transmitted _____7_____ respiratory droplets and airborne particles," Torres explained. "Therefore, it makes sense that these _____8_____ measures are also working against other respiratory viruses."

_____9_____ the future, Torres advises maintaining these measures. "If we continue to be vigilant and use these measures, we could have a _____10_____ flu season this year," he said. "This could be a 'silver lining' to the social distancing measures we have implemented to fight COVID-19."

1. A. design   B. designed   C. to design   D. designing
2. A. reducing   B. encouraging   C. ignoring   D. exaggerating
3. A. uncontrollable   B. inactive   C. uncommon   D. prevalent
4. A. more   B. much   C. fewer   D. few
5. A. similar   B.dissimilar   C. poor   D. good
6. A. coincidental   B. ironic   C. remarkable   D. unexpected
7. A. by   B. through   C. to   D. from
8. A. experimental   B. social   C. preventative   D. political
9. A. Looking up   B. Looking to   C. Looking for   D. Looking through
10. A. typical   B. severe   C. unexpected   D. mild

III. Translation

Directions: *Translate the following passage into Chinese.*

CDC also recommends prompt treatment with influenza antiviral medication for people who have flu or suspected flu and are experiencing severe illness (such as being hospitalized) or are at higher risk of serious flu-related complications. When treatment is started within two days of developing flu symptoms, antiviral drugs can effectively reduce fever and flu symptoms, shortening the duration of illness by approximately one day. Moreover, they may decrease the risk of certain complications, such as ear infections in children, respiratory complications requiring antibiotics, and hospitalization in adults. It's important to note that antiviral drugs are not available over the counter and can only be obtained with a prescription from a healthcare provider.

recommend [ˌrekəˈmend]	**v.**建议，劝告；推荐，介绍
prompt [prɒmpt]	**adj.**迅速的，立刻的；及时的，准时的
antiviral medication	抗病毒药物
suspected [səˈspektɪd]	**adj.**有嫌疑的，疑似…的
complication [ˌkɒmplɪˈkeɪʃ(ə)n]	**n.**使复杂化的难题（或困难）；并发症
antibiotic [ˌæntibaɪˈɒtɪk]	**n.**抗生素，抗菌素
health care provider	医疗服务人员

IV. Writing

Directions: *You are to write on the topic "**The Impact of Electronic Products on Our Daily Lives**". You should base your composition on the Chinese outline given below and your essay should not be less than 100 words.*

1. 电子产品对我们日常生活的影响。

2. 电子产品的优点和缺点。

3. 如何合理使用电子产品？

Grammar Focus

★ 时态

英语语法中的时态（tense）是一种动词形式，不同的时态表示行为、动作和状态在不同的时间条件下发生或存在。因此，当我们说时态结构的时候，指的是相应时态下的动词形式。

英语时态分为 16 种：一般现在时、一般过去时、一般将来时、过去将来时，以及这四者的进行时、完成时和完成进行时，如下表所示（以 do 为例）。

	一般	完成	进行	完成进行
现在	现在一般时 do	现在完成时 have done	现在进行时 is doing	现在完成进行时 have been doing
过去	过去一般时 did	过去完成时 had done	过去进行时 was doing	过去完成进行时 had been doing

（续表）

	一般	完成	进行	完成进行
将来	将来一般时 will do	将来完成时 will have done	将来进行时 will be doing	将来完成进行时 will have been doing
过去将来	过去将来一般时 would do	过去将来完成时 would have done	过去将来进行时 would be doing	过去将来完成进行时 would have been doing

常见的几种英语时态结构及用法如下。

一、一般现在时（do/does, is/am/are）

一般现在时表示通常性、规律性、习惯性、真理性的动作或状态。

1、表现在还存在的习惯或规律，尤其与频率副词 every day、always、never、seldom 等连用。

例如：I usually get up late.

She keeps a diary every day.

2、表示人或事物的特点，现在的状态。

例如：He looks young.

We are students.

3、表示真理、事实、格言，即使出现在过去的语境中，仍用一般现在时。

例如：There are seven days in a week.

I learned that the sun and the earth attract each other when I was young.

4、表示一个按规定、计划或安排要发生的动作。（常用于列车、客车、飞机或轮船时刻表）。

例如：The plane arrives at six tomorrow.

The next train leaves at 3 o'clock this afternoon.

5、表将来状况，从句使用一般现在时，主句使用一般将来时。

例如：The more weakness you show, the more aggressive others will be.

If it rains tomorrow, we will stay at home.

二、一般过去时（did,was/were）

一般过去时表示过去某个时间里发生的动作或状态，或者表示过去习惯性、经常性的动作、行为。

1、表示过去某个时间发生的动作或情况。

例如：I bought some fruits yesterday.

2、表示过去习惯性动作。

would/ used to do 过去常常…

例如：The old man would sit on a bench in the quiet park and look at others for hours without doing anything or talking to anybody.

He used to visit his mother once a week.

三、一般将来时

一般将来时表示将来某个时间里将要发生的动作或状态，或者表示将来经常、反复发生的动作或行为。

1、基本结构是 will do

例如：We will send her a glass hand-made craft as her birthday gift.

2、表示"打算…，要…"时，可用 am/is/are going to do。

例如：This is just what I am going to say.

3、表示"即将、正要"时，可用 am/is/are about to do，强调近期内或马上要做的事。

例如：Don't worry, I am about to make a close examination on you.

4、"be to do"的两种用法

（1）表示"按计划、安排即将发生某事或打算做某事"。

例如：The professor is to be seen in the lab on Monday.

（2）该做或不该做的事情（语气上接近于 should、must、ought to、 have to），表示一种命令、规劝性语气。

例如：You are to go to bed and keep quiet, kids. Our guests are arriving in less than 10 minutes.

四、现在进行时（am,is,are doing）

现在进行时表示正在进行的动作或状态。

1、表示此时此刻正在发生的事情。

例如：He is listening to the music now.

2、表示目前一段时间内一直在做的事情，但不一定此时此刻正在做。

例如：I am studying computer this term.

3、现在进行时可以表示将来的含义，瞬时动词的进行一定表将来。

例如：I am leaving.

持续动词的进行只有将来的时间状语或有将来语境才表将来。

例如：I am travelling next month.

4、现在进行时与频度副词连用，表示说话者或褒义或贬义的感情色彩。

例如：He is always helping others.（褒义）

五、现在完成时（have,has done）

现在完成时表示某个动作或状态已经完成，并且该动作或状态对现在仍有影响或结果。

1、表示动作到现在为止已经完成或刚刚完成，强调对现在产生的影响。

例如：I bought a new house, but I haven't sold my old one yet, so at the moment I have two houses.

2、表示从过去某时刻开始，持续到现在的动作或情况，并且有可能会继续延续下去。此时经常用延续性动词。

时间状语常用 since 加一个过去的时间点，或 for 加一段时间，或 by 加一个现在时间。

例如：Great as Newton was, many of his ideas have been challenged today and are being modified by the work of scientists of our time.

六、过去进行时（was,were doing）

过去进行时表示在过去某个时间点或时间段内正在发生的动作，强调动作的持续性和正在进行。

1、表示在过去一个具体的时间正在发生的动作。

例如：Mary was listening to light music 10 minutes ago.

2、表示过去某个时间段内一直在发生的事情。

例如：I was travelling in London last summer vacation.

3、过去进行时可以表示过去将来的含义。

瞬时动词的过去进行时一定表示过去将来的含义。

例如：Then she said she was leaving.

持续动词的过去进行时只有在有过去将来的时间状语或过去将来的语境下才能表示过去将来。

例如：She said that she was travelling the next day.

4、过去进行时和频度副词连用可以表示说话者或褒义或贬义的感情色彩。

例如：When he lived in country，he was always helping the poor.

七、过去完成时（had done）

过去完成时表示在过去某个时间之前已经完成的动作或状态。

1、表示在过去的某个时间或动作以前已经完成的动作或已经存在的状态，即 "过去的过去"。

例如：Until then, his family hadn't heard from him for six months.

2、表示从过去的过去开始，持续到过去的动作或情况，并且有可能会继续延续下去，此时经常用延续性动词。

例如：By the time I left the school, he had taught the class for 3 years.

八、过去将来进行时（would be doing）

过去将来进行时表示从过去的某个时间看将要发生的事。

例如：The government promised that a new highway would be being built next July.

Have a check on your grammar 过关演练

Directions: Choose the best answer to complete the sentence.

1. I _____ a book about China last week. I _____ it very much.

A. bought, liked

B. have bought, like

C. am buying, like

D. will buy, have liked

2. By the time you _____ this message, I _____ already left for the airport.

A. read, will

B. are reading, have

C. will read, have

D. have read, will have

3. My sister _____ piano lessons since she was six years old.

A. takes　　　　B. took　　　　C. has been taking　　　D. had taken

4. If it _____ tomorrow, we will cancel the picnic.

A. rains　　　　B. is raining　　　C. will rain　　　　D. would rain

5. He _____ to Paris three times before he finally decided to settle down there.

A. goes　　　　B. went　　　　C. has gone　　　　D. had gone

Unit Four   Food and Health

Listening & Speaking

Role-play

Listen to the following conversations, and play the role with your partner.

Dialogue One

Doctor: What seems to be the problem?

Patient: I got indigestion.

Doctor: How does the indigestion affect you?

Patient: All the food stays up here. (pointing to the chest)

Doctor: When does it occur?

Patient: Three to four hours after a meal.

Doctor: What is it like? A pain?

Patient: Yes, a pain.

Doctor: What kind? Burning, stabbing?

Patient: It feels like there is some wind there, and I want to get rid of it.

Doctor: Do you burp?

Patient: Not much.

Doctor: Does it bother you at night?

Patient: No.

Doctor: Does it occur when you're hungry?

Patient: Yes, I have a severe pain in my stomach, and I feel like I'll collapse if I don't eat right away.

Doctor: How is your appetite?

Patient: Not good.

Doctor: Has it always been poor?

Patient: No, it started to deteriorate ten years ago.

Doctor: Has it changed much in the last few months?

Patient: I think the medicine must push the food down and then I feel hungry.

Doctor: You'd better take some tests. I will prescribe some medicine for you after examination.

Dialogue Two

Doctor: Hello, I'm Dr. Johnson. What can I do for you today?

Woman: Hi, Dr. Johnson. I've been struggling with my weight, and I've noticed some changes in my health that worry me.

Doctor: I appreciate you reaching out. Let's discuss your weight and any specific concerns you have.

Woman: I've been overweight for a while, and lately, I've been feeling fatigued, experiencing joint pain, and having difficulty with simple physical activities.

Doctor: Thank you for sharing that. Your health is a priority, and we can work on addressing these issues. I'd like to run some tests to better understand your overall health and discuss potential lifestyle changes.

Woman: I'm willing to do whatever it takes to improve my health. What kind of tests do you recommend?

Doctor: We'll start with a basic physical examination and some blood tests to check cholesterol, blood sugar, and other relevant factors. Additionally, we may consider imaging tests if needed.

Woman: Sounds good. What about my weight? I've tried diets before, but nothing seems to work for long.

Doctor: Weight management is a gradual process, and we'll focus on sustainable changes. I'll recommend a balanced diet and regular physical activity tailored to your needs. We can also explore any underlying factors that might be contributing to your weight.

Woman: I appreciate your guidance, Dr. Johnson. I'm ready to make positive changes for my health.

Doctor: That's a positive mindset. We'll take it step by step, and I'm here to support you on this journey. If you have any questions or concerns along the way, don't hesitate to reach out.

Woman: Thank you, Dr. Johnson. I'm looking forward to improving my health with your help.

Speaking Practice

Fill in each blank with the choice that best suits the situation until the dialogue is complete. Then play the role with your partner.

Dialogue One

Doctor: Good morning! What seems to be the problem?

Man: Good morning, doctor. I've been having really bad diarrhea in the past two days, _____1_____

Doctor: I see. I'll ask you a few questions to understand it better. Have you experienced any other symptoms like stomach cramps, fever, or nausea?

Man: Yeah, I've had stomach cramps, and I felt a bit feverish yesterday, but it's gone now.

Doctor: Thank you for sharing that. It could be an infection or something you ate. _____2_____ and we might need a stool sample to determine the cause.

Man: Okay, I'm willing to accept any help, I just want this to come to an end.

Doctor: I understand. In the meantime, focus on staying hydrated with water, electrolyte drinks, and eat bland, easy-to-digest foods. Avoid dairy, spicy, and greasy foods for now.

Man: Got it. How long do you think it will take for the medication to work?

Doctor: _____3_____ If the symptoms persist or worsen, come back for a follow-up. And remember, if you notice any signs of dehydration, such as excessive thirst or dark urine, seek medical attention immediately.

Man: Thanks, doctor. I'll follow your advice.

Doctor: You're welcome. Take care, and I hope you feel better soon. If you have any concerns, don't hesitate to contact us.

A. It varies, but you should start feeling better in a day or two.

B. You'll be fine soon.

C. I'll prescribe some medication to help with the symptoms.

D. and it doesn't seem to be getting better.

Dialogue Two

Nurse: Good morning, Mr. Zhang. How are you feeling today?

Patient: Good morning, Miss Chen. I feel great!

Nurse: Good._____4_____ How does it sound?

Patient: Fantastic, I'm really looking forward to going home.

Nurse: Mr. Zhang, you will need to continue following a low-salt diet even after you leave the hospital.

Patient: Why do I need to continue doing that?

Nurse: You still have high blood pressure, and excessive salt can worsen it.
_____5_____

Patient: I refrain from adding salt to my food now.

Nurse: That's good. Many foods contain salt. Here is a list of foods you should avoid.

Patient: I didn't know that onion has salt in it.

Nurse: Well, please check the labels first. Here is an explanation of your new medicine. It is a diuretic that means it will make you urinate more. This will help your blood pressure under control. However, the medication may lead to potassium loss, _____6_____

Patient: Like bananas?

Nurse: Exactly, there is a list of foods that have potassium.

Patient: Thank you very much.

Nurse: You are welcome! Feel free to ask me any questions whenever you have them.

A. Don't mention it, it's my job.

B. You can be discharged tomorrow.

C. So, it's important to eat foods rich in potassium.

D. So, you should be cautious about consuming salt or sodium.

Dialogue Three

David: Hey, have you ever thought about the importance of developing good eating habits?

Mark: Yeah, I guess it's important, but I never really paid much attention to it.

David: Well, _____7_____ It affects our energy levels, mood, and even how well we sleep.

Mark: Really? I never realized it could have such a big impact.

David: Absolutely. A balanced diet with plenty of fruits, vegetables, whole grains, and lean proteins provides essential nutrients that our bodies need to function properly.

Mark: But it's so hard to resist all those tempting snacks and fast food.

David:_____8_____ But developing good eating habits doesn't mean giving up everything you love. It's about moderation and making healthier choices most of the time.

Mark: I suppose that makes sense. Where should I start?

David: Start by adding more fruits and vegetables to your meals, they're packed with vitamins and minerals. _____9_____

Mark: I do tend to have a sweet tooth. Any alternatives?

David: Opt for natural sweeteners like honey or choose fresh fruits when you're craving something sweet. And don't forget to drink plenty of water throughout the day.

Mark: Water instead of soda? That's a big change.

David: It is, but your body will thank you for it. _____ 10 _____

Mark: I guess I never really considered all these benefits. Thanks for the advice.

David: No problem! Small changes can lead to big improvements in your health over time. In addition, you'll likely feel more energized and focused.

A. It can be a challenge.

B. Water is crucial for digestion, metabolism, and overall hydration.

C. And try to cut back on sugary drinks and processed snacks.

D. what we eat plays a huge role in our health.

Reading & Writing

Text A

Hot Drinks and Cancer Risk

Next time you make yourself a hot cup of tea or coffee, you might want to let it cool down a bit before taking a sip.

Researchers say letting your hot drinks cool off could help you avoid some kinds of cancer. In fact, the United Nations' cancer research agency decided to list hot drinks with lead, gasoline and exhaust fumes as "possibly carcinogenic". In other words, each one could cause cancer.

The International Agency for Research on Cancer (IARC) is part of the World Health Organization (WHO). The IARC released its discoveries in the medical journal Lancet Oncology. According to IARC researchers, there is evidence suggesting that consuming beverages at temperatures exceeding 65 degrees Celsius may lead to esophageal cancer. The team analyzed results from studies conducted in Iran, China, and South America, where tea and coffee were frequently served at temperatures of 70 degrees Celsius or higher.

In developed countries, health experts have linked esophageal cancer to smoking and alcoholic consumption. Nevertheless, this type of cancer is more prevalent in regions where people drink beverages at very high temperatures.

In Europe and the United States, a significant number of individuals prefer their coffee and tea at temperatures approximately 60 degrees Celsius, often with the addition of milk, effectively reducing the temperature. However, tea-drinkers in Iran and South America often enjoy their beverages at closer to 70 degrees Celsius. The researchers note that South Americans not only drink tea at high temperatures but also utilize a metal straw, delivering the heated liquid directly into the throat.

The findings, however, are good news for coffee drinkers. In 1991, the World Health Organization listed coffee as "possibly carcinogenic". WHO officials have since changed their position on that listing. They now suggest that the temperature of your hot drink is a greater risk factor than the actual drink itself. Drinking very hot beverages is one probable cause of esophageal cancer and it is the temperature, <u>rather than</u> the drinks themselves, that may work.

The Coffee Association called the change "great news for coffee drinkers". However, the prevalence of esophageal cancer is worth noting. Globally, it ranks as the eighth most common cancer, claiming approximately 400,000 lives in 2012.

(371 words)

New Words

cancer ['kænsə(r)]	**n.**癌；癌症；邪恶；毒瘤
lead [li:d , led]	**n.** 铅；领先的地位；线索；主角；导线
	v.在…前面走；引路；领导；导致；引导；过（某种生活）
gasoline ['gæsəli:n , ˌgæsə'li:n]	**n.**汽油
carcinogenic [ˌkɑ:sɪnə'dʒenɪk]	**adj.**致癌的
release [rɪ'li:s]	**v.**公布；释放；松开；发泄；解雇；（使）放松
	n.释放；发行；排放；解脱
evidence ['evɪdəns]	**n.**证据；（法庭）证物，证词
	v.证明
beverage ['bevərɪdʒ]	**n.** 饮料
exceed [ɪk'si:d]	**v.**超过；超越
esophageal [i:ˌsɒfə'dʒi:əl]	**adj.**食道的，食管的
analyze ['ænəlaɪz]	**v.**分析；分解；化验
alcoholic [ˌælkə'hɒlɪk]	**adj.**（含）酒精的；饮酒引起的
	n.酒鬼，嗜酒如命的人
prevalent ['prevələnt]	**adj.**流行的，盛行的；普遍存在的，普遍发生的
significant [sɪg'nɪfɪkənt]	**adj.**重要的；显著的；意味深长的
approximately [ə'prɒksɪmətli]	**adv.**大约；近似
utilize ['ju:təlaɪz]	**vt.**利用，使用
official [ə'fɪʃl]	**n.**官员；裁判员
	adj.官方的；公务的；公开的；公务的；冠冕堂皇的

association [əˌsəʊsiˈeɪʃn]	**n.**协会，联盟；关系；联系，联想；因果关系
worth [wɜːθ]	**adj.**价值，值…钱；值得；拥有…价值的财产
	n.价值，意义，作用

Phrases & Expressions

cool down	（使）变凉；冷静下来；消气；降温
take a sip	尝一口；小啜；喝一小口
exhaust fumes	排出的废气
in other words	换句话说
World Health Organization (WHO)	世界卫生组织（世卫组织）
degree Celsius	摄氏度（℃）
lead to	导致
not only… but also…	不仅…还…
rather than	而不是
be worth doing…	值得做…

Reading Comprehension

Directions: *Choose the best answer to each of the following questions.*

1. According to the passage, what did the United Nations' cancer research agency list as "possibly carcinogenic" along with hot drinks? _____

A. Lead

B. Gasoline

C. Exhaust fumes

D. All of the above

2. In which medical journal did the IARC publish their findings? _____

A. Journal of Medicine and Health

B. Lancet Oncology

C. Cancer Research Journal

D. International Journal of Scientific Studies

3. What temperature range, as mentioned in the passage, is associated with a potential risk of esophageal cancer when consuming hot beverages? _____

A. Below 60 degrees Celsius

B. Between 60 and 65 degrees Celsius

C. Exceeding 65 degrees Celsius

D. Below 70 degrees Celsius

4　What factors are commonly linked to esophageal cancer in developed countries, according to the passage? _____

A. High-temperature beverage consumption

B. Smoking and alcoholic consumption

C. Adding milk to hot drinks

D. Metal straw usage

5. According to the passage, why did the World Health Organization (WHO) change its position on coffee's classification as "possibly carcinogenic"? _____

A. Due to new evidence proving coffee's safety

B. Because of increased coffee consumption worldwide

C. The focus shifted from the drink itself to its temperature

D. Pressure from the National Coffee Association

Text B

A Healthy Diet Blueprint: Path to Well-Being

It's important for you to eat right in order to energize your body for the demanding aspects of your life — whether it's studying, working, or some recreational activities.

You may feel like you don't have time to eat right or perhaps you're uncertain about the concept of eating well. The most common mistakes include insufficient consumption of fruits, vegetables, and high-fiber foods, coupled with excessive intake of fried foods, junk foods, sugary snacks, and sodas.

Healthy eating is not about strict dietary restrictions, aiming for an unrealistic thinness, or denying yourself the pleasure of the foods you enjoy. Instead, it's about experiencing positive well-being, increasing energy, enhancing health, and maintaining a more stable mood. If you feel overwhelmed by all the contradictory nutrition advice and diet recommendations out there, you're not alone, because it appears common that some experts advocate for a particular food while others suggest the opposite. However, by selectively following these simple tips, you can navigate through the confusion and discover how to create a tasty, varied, and nutritious diet that benefits both your mind and body.

Maintaining a healthy diet involves achieving a proper balance of essential nutrients through the consumption of beneficial foods such as vegetables, fruits, grains, meats, etc.

What positive effects can maintaining a healthy diet have on your mood?

While it's common knowledge that maintaining a proper diet supports weight management and prevents certain health issues, it also significantly influences your mood and overall well-being. Research indicates a connection between consuming a typical Western diet—characterized by processed meats, packaged meals, takeout food, and sugary snacks—and elevated occurrences of depression, stress, <u>bipolar disorder</u>, and anxiety. Moreover, an unhealthy diet might <u>contribute to</u> the onset of mental health disorders like ADHD, Alzheimer's disease, and schizophrenia, <u>as well as</u> an elevated risk of suicide among young individuals.

Increasing the consumption of fresh fruits and vegetables, preparing meals in your own kitchen, and decreasing the intake of sugar and refined carbohydrates can potentially enhance mood and decrease the likelihood of mental health issues. If you have already been diagnosed with a mental health problem, adopting a healthy diet can even help to manage your symptoms and regain control of your life.

What defines a healthy diet?

Maintaining a healthy diet doesn't have to be overly complex. Although certain foods or nutrients are known to positively impact mood, the crucial factor is your overall dietary pattern. The key to a healthy diet should involve <u>substituting</u> processed foods <u>with</u> whole, natural alternatives whenever you can. Consuming foods in a state that closely resembles how they are found in nature can significantly influence your mental, physical, and emotional well-being.

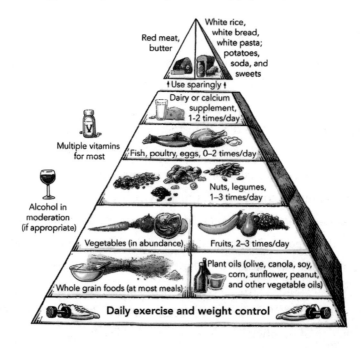

The Harvard Healthy Eating Pyramid reflects the latest advancements in nutritional science. The broad base represents the most crucial elements, with the narrower top indicating foods that should be consumed sparingly or avoided altogether. It emphasizes the importance of daily exercise and weight control in the broadest and most significant category. Fats from healthy sources, like plants, are situated in the wider section of the pyramid, while refined carbohydrates such as white bread and white rice are placed at the narrow top. Red meat is advised in moderation, while fish, poultry, and eggs are recommended as healthier options.

(547 words)

New Words

blueprint [ˈbluːprɪnt]	**n.**蓝图，设想；（基因）模型
energize [ˈenədʒaɪz]	**v.**加强，给…以活力；使活跃
insufficient [ˌɪnsəˈfɪʃnt]	**adj.**不足的，不够的；绌；亏短；支绌
intake [ˈɪnteɪk]	**n.**摄入，摄取；吸入，进气
well-being [ˈwel biːɪŋ]	**n.**健康；安乐
stable [ˈsteɪbl]	**adj.**稳定的；持重的；牢固的
overwhelmed [ˌəʊvəˈwelmd]	**adj.**不知所措的，被淹没的；被压倒的
nutrition [njuˈtrɪʃn]	**n.**营养
specific [spəˈsɪfɪk]	**adj.**独特的；明确的
advocate [ˈadvəkeɪt]	**vt.**拥护；主张；鼓吹
	n.拥护者，支持者；辩护律师
navigate [ˈnævɪgeɪt]	**v.**导航，确定路线；航行；驾驭，成功应付（困难处境）
confusion [kənˈfjuːʒn]	**n.**困惑；混淆；尴尬；混乱局面
nutrient [ˈnjuːtriənt]	**n.**营养物，营养品，养分，养料；滋养物
beneficial [ˌbenɪˈfɪʃl]	**adj.**有益的，有帮助的
indicate [ˈɪndɪkeɪt]	**v.**表明，暗示；指示；象征；
typical [ˈtɪpɪkl]	**adj.**典型的；特有的；一贯的，平常的
characterize [ˈkærəktəraɪz]	**v.**使具有特点；是…的特征；描绘
occurrence [əˈkʌrəns]	**n.**发生，出现；遭遇，事件
onset [ˈɒnset]	**n.** [医]发病；攻击，袭击；开始
schizophrenia [ˌskɪtsəˈfriːniə]	**n.** [医]精神分裂症；矛盾
enhance [ɪnˈhɑːns]	**v.**提高，增强；改进
decrease [dɪˈkriːs , ˈdiːkriːs]	**v.**减少
	n.减少

likelihood [ˈlaɪklihʊd]	**n.**可能，可能性
diagnose [ˈdaɪəgnəʊz]	**v.**诊断；判断
adopt [əˈdɒpt]	**v.**采用；领养；正式通过
symptom [ˈsɪmptəm]	**n.**症状；征兆
regain [rɪˈgeɪn]	**v.**复得，重回；回收；恢复（失物、失地、健康等）
define [dɪˈfaɪn]	**v.**阐明；限定；给…下定义；描出…的界线
impact [ˈɪmpækt , ɪmˈpækt]	**n.**影响；作用；冲击力
	v.对…有影响；冲击；撞击
crucial [ˈkruːʃl]	**adj.**至关重要的，关键性的
alternative [ɔːlˈtɜːnətɪv]	**n.**可供选择的事物
	adj.替代的，备选的；另类的
resemble [rɪˈzembl]	**v.**像；类似
reflect　[rɪˈflekt]	**v.**反映；反射；照出（影像）；沉思；表达
represent [ˌreprɪˈzent]	**v.**代表；象征；维护…的利益；正式提出
sparingly [ˈspeərɪŋlɪ]	**adv.**缺少地；节约地；保守地；仁慈地
emphasize [ˈemfəsaɪz]	**v.**强调；重视；使突出
category [ˈkætəgəri]	**n.**种类；类别
moderation [ˌmɒdəˈreɪʃn]	**n.**自我节制；适度；稳定，镇定
option [ˈɒpʃn]	**n.**选择；选择权；可选择的事物

Phrases & Expressions

coupled with	加上，外加
dietary restriction	饮食限制，[医]食谱限制
aim for	计划，打算
refined carbohydrates	精制碳水化合物
achieve a proper balance	达到一个适当的平衡
bipolar disorder	双相障碍；双相型障碍
as well as	和…一样；除…以外还；既…又；和，以及
substitute…with	用…代替

Reading Comprehension

Directions: *Choose the best answer to each of the following questions.*

1. According to the passage, what are some common mistakes in diet? _____

A. Insufficient consumption of fruits and vegetables

B. Excessive intake of unhealthy foods

C. Eating too much healthy foods

D. Both A and B

2. What is the suggestion about dealing with conflicting nutrition advice in this passage?

_____

A. Ignoring all advice

B. Following the advice of one expert

C. Navigating through the confusion with some simple tips

D. Avoiding any dietary changes

3. According to the passage, how should people do to manage the symptoms of a mental

health problem? _____

A. More exercises will help

B. Following a healthy diet can work

C. More meats and grains will cure

D. Sleeping well is a solution

4. According to the passage, what does a healthy diet involve? _____

A. Exclusively consuming processed foods

B. Achieving a proper balance of essential nutrients

C. Strict dietary restrictions

D. Ignoring overall dietary patterns

5. How does the Harvard Healthy Eating Pyramid emphasize the importance of exercise

and weight control? _____

A. Placing them at the narrow top

B. Excluding them from the pyramid

C. Positioning them in the broadest category

D. Ignoring their relevance

Language Practice

I. Vocabulary and Structure

Directions: *Choose the one that best completes the sentence.*

1. The detective needed to _____ the evidence carefully to solve the complex case.

A. analyze   B. analysis   C. analytical   D. analogy

2. The journey took _____ eight hours.

A. scarcely   B. overly   C. particularly   D. approximately

3. These prejudices are particularly _____ among people living in the South.

A. crucial   B. significant   C. prevalent   D. beneficial

4. The book is worth _____.

A. read   B. to read   C. reading   D. have read

5. Her achievements have _____ our expectations.

A. expressed   B. exceeded   C. expected   D. experienced

6. The higher the tree is, the _____ the wind is.

A. strongest   B. stronger   C. strong   D. strongly

7. Pulse can _____ at any place where there is a large artery.

A. measure   B. have measured   C. measuring   D. be measured

8. Anson was always speaking highly of his role in the play,_____ made the others unhappy.

A. which   B. how   C. what   D. who

9. At present, a large number of women, especially those from the countryside, _____ for the clothing industry.

A. work   B. works   C. working   D. worked

10. Scarcely _____ when it began to snow.

A. the game had started   B. did the game start

C. had the game started   D. the game started

11. They are accustomed _____ late on weekends.

A. of sleeping   B. to sleeping   C. for sleeping   D. at sleeping

12. If you want to buy this dress, you'd better _____ first to make sure it fits you.

A. take it off   B. tidy it up   C. try it on   D. pay for it

13. We do our best for our dreams together and a small success can give us a sense of _____.

A. responsibility   B. entertainment   C. amusement   D. achievement

14. — Excuse me, is the park far from here?

— No, it's about _____.

A. 10 minutes walk   B. 10 minute's walk

C. 10 minute walk   D. 10 minutes' walk

15. — To go abroad or not after graduation, it's a question.

— You may take _____ of the roads, but being home in the end matters.

A. both   B. either   C. neither   D. none

16. — Excuse me, do you know _____? The train has just left.

— Yes. The next train will arrive in half an hour.

A. if there will be another train   B. how can I get to the train station

C. how much a ticket costs   D. how far is it from here

17. —_____ fast China is developing!

— Yes, we are so lucky to live in such great country.

A. How   B. What   C. How a   D. What a

18. Fossils are the evidence of past life _____ in the rocks of the Earth's crust.

A. prepared   B. proposed   C. postponed   D. preserved

19. The speaker tried her best to make herself _____ in spite of so much noise.

A. hear   B. be heard   C. heard   D. hearing

20. Jessica was assigned to _____ the HR Department.

A. take advantage of   B. take charge of   C. take care of   D. take control of

II. Cloze

Directions: *Choose the best one to complete the passage.*

The history of tea in China is long and complex. Chinese people have been drinking tea for ____1____. Scholars hold tea in high esteem because of its therapeutic effects in treating various ailments. Among the nobility, the consumption of high-quality tea is considered as a symbol of their social status. Meanwhile, the common people's love for tea is purely based on their enjoyment of its flavor. In *The Divine Farmer's Herb-Root Classic*, the legendary emperor Shennong asserted that tea infusions had therapeutic benefits for various conditions, including tumors, abscesses, bladder issues, and lethargy. While the majority of health studies focus on green tea, there have also been investigations into other types, ____2____ black, oolong, and Pu'er tea.

Green tea ____3____ the highest medicinal value and the lowest caffeine content among all types of Chinese tea. Over the centuries, Chinese green tea has been associated ____4____ many health benefits, including cancer prevention. ____5____, green tea can increase the blood flow throughout the body. As a result, drinking green tea helps strengthen the blood vessels that provide oxygen and valuable nutrients to the heart and brain. Studies indicate that men who ____6____ consume Chinese green tea have a 75 percent lower likelihood of experiencing a stroke compared to those who do not drink this tea.

Many ancient writings and renowned books in Chinese history have ____7____ the health benefits and medicinal use of Pu'er tea. Pu'er tea is strongly believed to have a wide range of health benefits, including anti-aging effects, heart disease and cancer prevention, diabetes management, promotion of digestion and weight loss, enhancement of eyesight, improvement of blood circulation, and revival of individuals excessively intoxicated with alcohol. In many traditional Chinese restaurants, especially those known for serving dim sum, Pu'er tea is the customary drink provided. Its ability to effectively _____8_____ oily and fatty foods, aiding in digestion, makes it an ideal drink to accompany delicious Chinese dishes that often high in fat.

Although drinking tea has many benefits, consuming excessively strong tea can have _____9_____ effects on the body. Therefore, it is advisable to drink tea in _____10_____.

1. A. milestone   B. millionaire   C. millennia   D. military
2. A. such that   B. such as   C. just as   D. just about
3. A. possess   B. possessed   C. possessing   D. possesses
4. A. to   B. at   C. in   D. with
5. A. In addition   B. In a word   C. In advance   D. in case
6. A. seldom   B. regularly   C. never   D. scarcely
7. A. documented   B. document   C. documentary   D. documentation
8. A. bread up   B. break out   C. break down   D. break in
9. A. positive   B. neutral   C. adverse   D. active
10. A. celebration   B. reputation   C. contribution   D. moderation

II. Translation

Directions: *Translate the following passage into Chinese.*

What is moderation? In essence, it entails consuming only the amount of food necessary for your body's requirements. The goal is to feel satisfied after a meal without being overly stuffed. For many of us, moderation means reducing our current food intake, but it doesn't mean giving up the foods we love. For example, having bacon for breakfast once a week can be considered moderation if it's followed by a healthy lunch and dinner, but not if it's followed by a box of donuts and a sausage pizza. Cooking more meals at home can help you take control of your diet and closely monitor the ingredients in your food. This not only results in consuming fewer calories but also helps you avoid the chemical additives, extra sugar, and unhealthy fats commonly found in packaged and takeout foods. Staying away from these elements can stop you from feeling tired, bloated, and irritable. Additionally, it can relieve symptoms related to depression, stress, and anxiety.

moderation [ˌmɒdəˈreɪʃn]	n. 适度；自我节制
In essence	本质上，大体上，其实

monitor ['mɒnɪtə(r)]	**v.** 监控；监听
result in	导致
chemical additives	化学添加剂
bloated ['bləʊtɪd]	**adj.** 发胀的
irritable ['ɪrɪtəbl]	**adj.** 易怒的，急躁的
relieve [rɪ'li:v]	**v.** 解除；缓解

IV. Writing

Directions: *You are to write on the topic "**My Way of Seeing Life**". You should base your composition on the Chinese outline given below and your essay should not be less than 100 words.*

1. 人们从不同的角度看待人生。
2. 我所推崇的看法。
3. 说明持这种看法的理由。

Grammar Focus

★ 非谓语动词

非谓语动词又称为非限定动词，指在句子中不是谓语的动词，即动词的非谓语形式，主要包括分词（现在分词和过去分词）、动名词和不定式三种形式，即 doing、done 和 to do。非谓语动词除了不能独立作谓语，可以承担句子的其他成分，如可以充当主语、宾语、状语等。

一、分词

1. 现在分词

现在分词既具有动词的一些特征，又具有形容词和副词的句法功能。

（1）作定语

In the <u>following</u> month, she worked even harder.

China is a <u>developing</u> country.

（2）作表语

The present situation is <u>encouraging</u>.

The story sounds very <u>moving</u>.

（3）作状语

<u>Walking in the street</u>, I met a friend of my mother. （时间状语）

<u>Being a league member</u>, he is always helping others. （原因状语）

Lucy sat at the table <u>reading China Daily</u>. （方式状语，表伴随）

She dropped the glasses, <u>breaking it into pieces</u>. （结果状语）

<u>Working hard</u>, you will do better in the final examination. （条件状语）

<u>Though raining heavily</u>, it cleared up very soon. （让步状语）

（4）作宾语补足语

现在分词常用在 see、watch、hear、feel、find、get、keep、notice、observe、listen to、look at 等后面作宾语补足语。

She <u>saw people coming and going.</u>

We <u>heard her singing</u> in the classroom.

They <u>kept the bus waiting</u> at the gate.

2. 过去分词

过去分词只有一种形式：规则动词由动词原形加词尾-ed 构成。不规则动词的过去分词没有统一的规则要求，要一一记住。

（1）作定语

Our class went on an <u>organized</u> trip last month.

Most of the people <u>invited</u> to the party were famous scientists.

（2）作表语

The cup is <u>broken</u>.

She looked <u>worried</u> after reading the letters.

（3）作状语

<u>Once seen</u>, it can never be forgotten. （时间状语）

<u>Confused by the stones</u> flying at them from all sides, the girls ran into the building. （原因状语）

<u>Given more time</u>, you will achieve success. （条件状语）

<u>Even though defeated again and again</u>, the athlete didn't give up. （让步状语）

（4）作宾语补足语

过去分词常用在 see、watch、hear、feel、find、get、keep、notice、observe、listen to、look at 等后面作宾语补足语。

When she got to school, she <u>saw the door locked.</u>

After waking up, he <u>found everyone gone.</u>

二、动词不定式（**to do**）

动词不定式具有名词、形容词、副词的特征。

1. 作主语

To give up smoking is necessary.

To lose your heart means failure.

2. 作表语

His job is to clean the room.

She appears to have caught a cold.

3. 作宾语

常与不定式作宾语连用的动词有 want、hope、wish、offer、fail、plan、learn、pretend、refuse、manage、help、agree、promise、prefer。如果不定式（宾语）后面有宾语补足语，则用 it 作形式宾语，真正的宾语（不定式）后置，放在宾语补足语后面。

David found it important to study the present situation.

4. 作宾语补足语

在复合宾语中，动词不定式可充当宾语补足语，以下动词常跟这种复合宾语 Want、wish、ask、tell、order、beg、permit、help、advise、persuade、allow、prepare、cause、force、call on、wait for、invite. 此外，介词有时也与这种复合宾语连用。

With a lot of work to do, she didn't go to the supermarket.

5. 作定语

The train to arrive is from Beijing.

Tom is the first student to come and the last to leave.

6. 作状语

Her parents worked day and night to get the money.（表目的）

They arrived late only to find the train had gone. （表结果）

Tracy was very happy to meet her old friends. （表原因）

The question is simple for her to answer. （表程度）

三、动名词

动名词既具有动词的一些特征，又具有名词的句法功能。

	主动	被动
一般式（与谓语动词同时发生）	doing	being done
完成式（与谓语动词发生之前）	having done	having been done

1. 作主语

Reading is an art.

<u>Using the right hand to shake hands</u> is a convention in many countries.

当动名词短语作主语时常用 it 作形式主语。

<u>It is no use</u> telling him not to worry.

2. 作表语

In the ant city, the queen's job is <u>laying eggs</u>.

My job is <u>teaching</u>.

3. 作宾语

（1）有些动词后面要求跟动名词作宾语，如 admit、excuse、anticipate、fancy、practice、deny、prevent、propose、finish、avoid、delay、appreciate、mind、 save、involve、imagine、permit、miss、recommend、enjoy 等。

Will you <u>admit having broken the window</u>?

I <u>recommend buying the novel</u>.

（2）有些动词短语后也要求跟动名词作宾语，如 can't help、feel like、give up、can't stand、look forward to、pay attention to、succeed in、be used to、object to、insist on、be engaged in、be worth、be fond of 等。

Do you <u>feel like having a cup of tea</u>?

Jason <u>was used to getting up early</u> on weekends.

（3）动名词作宾语时，若跟有宾语补足语，则常用形式宾语 it。

I found <u>it</u> no good making fun of others.

They consider <u>it</u> a waste of time arguing about it.

4. 作定语

There is a <u>swimming</u> pool.

He bought a <u>washing</u> machine last week.

5. 作同位语

His habit, <u>listening to the news</u> on the bus remains unchanged.

My job, <u>looking after these old people</u>, is rewarding.

Have a check on your grammar 过关演练

Directions: *Choose the best answer to complete the sentence.*

1. The play _____ next week aims mainly to reflect the local culture.

A. produced   B. being produced   C.to be produced   D. having been produced

2. _____ along the old Silk Road is an interesting and rewarding experience.

A. Travel   B. Travels   C. Traveled   D. Traveling

3. The meeting was put off because we _____ a meeting without Jack.

A. objected to having   B. objected to have

C. objected having   D. were objected to having

4. He walked along the street,_____ a song.

A. sing   B. sings   C. singing   D. sang

5. The house _____ last year will be pulled down.

A. built   B. was built   C. building   D. has been built

6. She can do what she can _____ the children in her neighborhood.

A. help   B. helps   C. helped   D. to help

7. We believe that AI _____ in many fields will _____ to help us solve many problems in the future.

A. is used, be used   B. is used, use

C. used, be used   D. used, use

8. They have no choice but _____ here.

A. to stay   B. staying   C. stayed   D. is staying

9. _____ his homework, he played football.

A. Have done   B. Having done   C. Done   D. Did

10. Lily took a taxi to the airport, only _____ her plane high up in the sky.

A. found   B. finding   C. being found   D. to find

Unit Five   Obesity

Listening & Speaking

Role-play

Listen to the following conversations, and play the role with your partner.

Dialogue One

Doctor: Good morning, madam.How can I help you?

Patient: Good morning. Doctor Smith.

Doctor: You must be Tracy. I saw that you scheduled this appointment a week ago.

Patient: That's right. Doctor.

Doctor: Take a seat, please. How was your diet?

Patient: Following your advice, I've lost 4 kg in the last two weeks.

Doctor: That's a marked improvement in your condition.

Patient: Well, I'm not coming here for my weight though.

Doctor: What's the matter?

Patient: I've recently been to the gyms for intensive exercises, but somehow I've got a pain in my shoulders!

Doctor: I'm sorry to hear that, Tracy. Remember that exercises are good for your health, but too much can lead to injuries.

Patient: Yeah, I want to lose weight as soon as possible.

Doctor: Rapid weight loss may not be the healthiest approach. I suggest taking a break from intense exercises while maintaining a balanced diet.

Patient: Alright, Doctor.

Doctor: I'll make a prescription for your ache.

Patient: Thank you, Doctor.

Dialogue Two

Andy: John, we are becoming fatter and fatter. It's high time we lost some weight.

John: I agree. Should we start to exercise more?

Andy: Absolutely. We should also focus on maintaining a healthy diet. I want to feel more confident about my body.

John: Me too. Have you heard of the Atkins diet? It's quite popular.

Andy: Rings a bell. What's it about?.

John: It's pretty famous. It focuses on restricting the amount of carbohydrates in your diet and replacing them with proteins and fats. The idea is that the absence of carbohydrates leads to your body burning fat for energy. It is great for losing weight.

Andy: Sounds good, but what about a vegan diet? No meat or animal products, supposedly beneficial for heart health.

John: It is, but some say it's not balanced. How about cutting out all processed foods and sticking to natural ones? It's said to be good both for weight loss and general health.

Andy: That one sounds appealing. Let's give it a try.

John: Okay, let's go for it!

Speaking Practice

Fill in each blank with the choice that best suits the situation until the dialogue is complete. Then play the role with your partner.

Dialogue One

Patient: I've been gaining weight recently. What can I do?

Doctor: Do you usually eat bread?

Patient: Yes, _____1_____.

Doctor: It would be beneficial if you substitute your regular bread with wholemeal bread. It has fewer calories and can also contribute to lowering your blood sugar.

Patient: Yes, _____2_____.

Doctor: Additionally, you should eat more leafy greens.

Patient: _____3_____

Doctor: Something like spinach would be good. They are rich in nutrients such as vitamin C, vitamin K, and vitamin A.

Patient: Normally, I seldom eat those greens. I will buy them on my way home.

A. I will keep that in mind.

B. Very often.

C. Thank you.

D. What kind of green leaves?

Dialogue Two

Mary: I can't continue this lifestyle anymore. _____4_____, I need to make a change.

Susan: Go for it. I support you. Do you have a plan on how to do it?

Mary: I already wrote a plan. I decided to lose weight safely and slowly.

Susan: _____5_____

Mary: Sure. I will work around 8 hours a day, spending 2 hours on meal preparation and 2 hours on exercise.

Susan: Wow, _____6_____

Mary: I've done some research on foods that are beneficial or harmful to health. I am heading to the store to buy them now. Would you like to go to the supermarket with me?

Susan: Of course, let's go together.

A. Does it hurt?

B. what a detailed plan!

C. Can I take a look at it?

D. From now on.

Dialogue Three

Mary: Let's start at the vegetable counter.

Susan: Sure. There are so many vegetables. _____7_____

Mary: We'll pick up spinach and broccoli.

Susan: Why those?

Mary: Because they have few calories and carbohydrates, but are rich in fiber, vitamins and minerals. That is very good for weight loss.

Susan: _____8_____ tomatoes and potatoes? Do you think we should buy them?

Mary: Tomatoes are very low in calories and high in fiber, so let's get those. But for potatoes, I think we should replace them with sweet potatoes.

Susan: _____9_____ Are white potatoes not good?

Mary: Sweet potatoes are lower in calories and keep you full longer.

Susan: You have researched very carefully.

Mary: Yep. We've got our vegetables. _____10_____.

Susan: People often eat avocados when losing weight, so, shall we buy some avocados?

Mary: Yes. I'm also thinking of picking up blueberries, strawberries and bananas.

Susan: Do these foods help with weight loss?

Mary: Yes. They all have a lot of vitamins and minerals.

A. Why?

B. Which ones should we get?

C. How about

D. Let's go to the fruit counter!

Reading & Writing

Text A

Obesity

Obesity has become a widespread global concern, affecting approximately 600 million people worldwide and increasing the risk of various health issues such as <u>heart disease</u>, stroke, and cancer. But in the 1970s and 1980s, experts began to question the extent to which obesity contributes to these disorders. Subsequent studies in the late 1990s and early 2000s revealed that some obese people led relatively healthy lives, giving rise to the concept of "<u>healthy obesity</u>", which gained value over the past 15 years, but scientists have recently questioned its existence. "Our new findings suggest that health measures may be necessary for all individuals with obesity, even those who were previously considered to be metabolically healthy, "says Mikael, "Since obesity is the major <u>gene expression</u> in fat cells, we should continue to <u>focus on</u> preventing obesity."

Medical professionals recognize obesity as a health issue, but they face challenges when addressing it with their patients. The results of two surveys — one involving primary care physicians and the other patients — indicate that, while most doctors express a desire to help patients <u>lose weight</u> and believe it is their responsibility, they often find it challenging to find suitable ways to initiate the conversation.

So while doctors may tell patients they are overweight, the conversation often ends there, said Christine C. Ferguson, director of <u>the Stop Obesity Alliance</u>. "Doctors don't feel they have good information to give. They felt they didn't have adequate tools to address this problem."

The lack of dialogue also negatively impacts patients. According to a survey involving more than 1,000 adults, the majority of overweight individuals are not aware of their weight status. Only 39 percent of surveyed overweight individuals had received information from a healthcare provider indicating that they were overweight.

Of those who were told they were obese, 90 percent were also told by their doctors to lose weight, the survey found. <u>In fact</u>, most have tried to lose weight and may have been successful <u>in the past</u> and many are still trying, the survey found. And many understand that losing even a small amount of weight can <u>have a positive impact on</u> their health and reduce their risk of obesity-related diseases like hypertension and diabetes.

Dr. William Bestermann Jr., medical director of <u>Holston Medical Group</u> in <u>Kingsport, Tennessee</u> — a city ranking 10th in obesity among metropolitan areas in the United States, emphasizes the importance of continuous dialogue on weight management. He stresses that the dialogue had to be an ongoing one and could not be dropped after just one mention of the problem. "If you're to be successful with helping your patients lose weight, you have to talk to them at actually every visit about their progress, and find something to encourage them and coach them." he said.

He acknowledged that many doctors tend to be not optimistic. "This is partly due to a prevalent belief, which doctors themselves may feel burdened by, that overweight people lack willpower, and engage in self-indulgence," he explained. "If doctors think this way, they may not spend time having a productive conversation."

(512 words)

New Words

obesity [əʊˈbiːsɪtɪ]	n.肥胖（症）
	adj. obese [əʊˈbiːs] 肥胖的；臃肿的
approximately [əˈprɒksɪmɪtlɪ]	adv.大概；大约
stroke [strəʊk]	n.（脑）卒中；中风
	v.轻抚；轻触
disorder [ˌdɪsˈɔːdə]	n.身体不适；失调
existence [ɪgˈzɪstəns]	n.实存；存在
measure [ˈmeʒə]	n.办法；措施；量度；测量工具
individual [ˌɪndɪˈvɪdʒʊəl]	n.（尤指有别于他人的）个人；个体
metabolically [ˌmetəˈbɒlɪklɪ]	adv.在新陈代谢方面；在代谢方面
gene [dʒiːn]	n.基因
survey [ˈsɜːveɪ]	n.综述；概况；概论；概略；调查
primary [ˈpraɪmərɪ]	adj.主要的；首要的；重要的
	n.居首位者；居于重要地位者
physician [fɪˈzɪʃən]	n.医生；（尤指）内科医生

responsibility [rɪˌspɒnsɪˈbɪlɪtɪ]	**n.**责任；（事故、过失等的）责任，罪责；职责
overweight [ˌəʊvəˈweɪt]	**n.**超重；过重；更重要
alliance [əˈlaɪəns]	**n** 结盟；联盟；同盟；（尤指军事的）盟约；结盟诸国
adequate [ˈædɪkwɪt]	**adj.**足够的；充足的；充分的；足够好的
address [əˈdres]	**v.**解决，处理；在…上写地址；向…说话；演讲
lack [læk]	**n.**缺乏；缺少；不足；没有；短缺的东西
	v.缺乏；需要
percent [pəˈsent]	**n.**百分比，百分数；百分之一
positive [ˈpɒzɪtɪv]	**adj.**积极的；乐观的；有建设性的；正面的
hypertension [ˌhaɪpəˈtenʃən]	**n.**高血压
diabetes[daɪəˈbiːtiːz]	**n.**糖尿病；多尿症；
metropolitan [ˌmetrəˈpɒlɪtn]	**adj.** 构成大城市的；大都会的；大城市的
ongoing [ˈɒnˌgəʊɪŋ]	**adj.**进行中的；不断发展的；持续存在的；
mention [ˈmenʃən]	**v.**（简短地）提及，说起
	n.提及；说到
coach [kəʊtʃ]	**n.**教练
	v.指导；训练；当…的教练；（尤指为帮助备考）辅导
acknowledge [əkˈnɒlɪdʒ]	**v.**承认；告知收到；确认收悉
optimistic[ˌɒptɪˈmɪstɪk]	**adj.**乐观的；乐观主义的
willpower[ˈwɪlˌpaʊə]	**n.**意志力；毅力；意念
self-indulgence[ˌself ɪnˈdʌldʒənt]	**n.** 任性，放纵
productive [prəˈdʌktɪv]	**adj.**富饶的；肥沃的；有生产力的

Phrases & Expressions

heart disease	心脏病
healthy obesity	健康性肥胖
gene expression	基因表达
focus on	集中注意力；关注
lose weight	减肥
in fact	事实上
in the past	在过去

have a positive impact on	对…有积极的影响
tend to	倾向于

Proper Names

the Stop Obesity Alliance	终止肥胖联盟
Holston Medical Group	霍尔斯顿医疗集团
Kingsport	金斯波特镇
Tennessee	田纳西州

Reading Comprehension

Choose the best answer to each of the following questions.

1. What is the primary global concern discussed in the passage? _____

A. Heart disease

B. Stroke

C. Cancer

D. Obesity

2. According to the passage, what concept gained prominence over the past 15 years but is now being questioned by scientists? _____

A. Healthy lifestyle

B. Healthy obesity

C. Metabolic health

D. Obesity prevention

3. How many of the patients surveyed have been advised by their doctors to lose weight? _____

A. About 350

B. About 390

C. About 900

D. About 1,000

4. What challenges do doctors face when addressing obesity with their patients, according to Christine C. Ferguson? _____

A. Lack of information

B. Inadequate tools

C. Unaware patients

D. Obesity-related tools

5. What does Dr. William Beckerman Jr. emphasize as crucial for successful weight management in patient? _____

    A. Onc-time conversation

    B. Regular and ongoing dialogue

    C. Lack of optimism

    D. Blaming patients for lack of willpower

Text B

Successful Weight Loss Plans

Obesity, also known as severe overweight, is a complex condition. Obesity in children and adolescents is rising at an alarming rate. Currently more than 15% of young people over the age of 6 are obese, with a rising trend also observed in those aged 5 and below. Too much television watching plays an important role in obesity in children. Not only is it a passive activity, but television also offers countless temptations（诱惑） with its advertisements for fast foods, sugar cereals, and unhealthy snacks. A study revealed that children who watched one hour or less of television per day had the lowest obesity rates, while those who watched four or more hours had the highest rates. Additionally, less physical exercise and increased sedentary activities are key factors in the prevalence of obesity among children. A high level of physical activity — not just using up energy — is crucial for weight control in young people.

A doctor may recommend medical interventions in addition to changes in behavior. However, according to experts, most effective weight-loss plans involve a well-balanced diet and regular exercise. People who want to avoid weight gain have to balance the number of calories they eat with the number of calories they use. To lose weight，you can reduce the number of calories you take in，or increase the number you use, or both. Experts at the National Institutes of Health suggest that for effective weight loss, people should engage in moderate or intensive physical exercise most days of the week, such as fast walking, sports or strength training.

A recent study at Stanford University analyzed four popular diet plans in the United States. Over three hundred overweight women, mostly in their thirties or forties, participated in the study, each following one of the four plans：Atkins，The Zone，Ornish or LEARN. The women attended diet classes and received written information about the food plans. At the end of a year，the women on the Atkins diet had lost the most，more than four and a half kilograms on average.

The research, conducted by Christopher Gardner and documented in the <u>Journal of the American Medical Association</u>, reveals that the Atkins diet may be more successful because of its simple message to lower the intake of sugar. Additionally，he noted that the advice to increase protein in the diet <u>leads to</u> more satisfying meals.

However, a recent report indicated that only a small number of people succeed in long-term dieting. Researchers at <u>the University of California</u> found that most dieters regained their lost weight within five years, often gaining even more. Conversely, those who successfully maintained their weight loss were generally individuals who incorporated regular exercise into their routine.

（464 words）

New Words

severe [sɪˈvɪə]	**adj.** 严厉的；苛刻的；朴素的；严厉的
complex[ˈkɒmpleks]	**adj.** 难懂的；复杂的；错综的
	n. 综合体；集合体；复合体；情结
adolescent [ˌædəˈlesnt]	**n.** 青少年
	adj. 青春期的；青少年期的；不成熟的；青涩的
alarming[əˈlɑːmɪŋ]	**adj.** 令人担忧的；使人惊恐的
currently[ˈkʌrəntlɪ]	**adv.** 目前；当前；眼下
passive [ˈpæsɪv]	**adj.** 顺从的；听之任之的；被动的；不动的
countless [ˈkaʊntlɪs]	**adj.** 无数的；数不尽的；不计其数的
temptation[tempˈteɪʃən]	**n.** 引诱；诱惑；诱惑物；有诱惑力的人
advertisement[ədˈvɜːtɪsmənt]	**n.** 广告；启事
cereal [ˈsɪərɪəl]	**n.** 谷类作物；谷类；谷物；（尤指早餐吃的）谷类食物
snack [snæk]	**n.** 点心，快餐；零食；一小口
	v. 吃点心；吃零食
significant [sɪgˈnɪfɪkənt]	**adj.** 可观的；相当大的；重要的
intervention[ˌɪntəˈvenʃən]	**n.** 调停；斡旋；干涉；干预；
behavior[bɪˈheɪvjə]	**n.** 行为，举止；态度；反应
well-balanced [ˈwelˈbælənst]	**adj.** 均衡的；搭配均衡的
avoid [əˈvɔɪd]	**v.** 避免；防止；戒绝；逃避
calorie [ˈkælərɪ]	**n.** 卡（路里）；小卡（热量单位）

moderate [ˈmɒdərɪt]	**adj.**温和的；不激进的；中等的；一般的
	n.温和派
intensive [ɪnˈtensɪv]	**adj.**加强的；强化的；集中的，密集的
diet [ˈdaɪət]	**n.**（尤指以控制体重为目的的）限制饮食，节食
kilogram[ˈkɪləgræm]	**n.**千克，公斤（国际单位制质量单位）
average [ˈævərɪdʒ]	**n.**一般量；平均值
	adj.平均的；典型的；一般的；中等的；平常的
intake [ˈɪnˌteɪk]	**n.**摄入物；摄入量；接收量；吸入；（流体的）入口
protein [ˈprəʊtiːn]	**n.**蛋白质

Phrases & Expressions

be known as	被称为
at a/an … rate	以某种速度
play an important role	扮演着重要的角色；起重要作用
take in	摄入
on a … diet	进行…饮食疗法
lead to	引发；导致

Proper Names

the National Institutes of Health	国立卫生研究院
Stanford University	斯坦福大学
Atkins	阿特金斯饮食法
The Zone	区域饮食法
Ornish	欧尼许饮食法
LEARN	LEARN 减肥法（分别代表 Lifestyle、Exercise、Attitudes、Relationships、Nutrition）
the Journal of the American Medical Association	美国医学会杂志
the University of California	（美国）加州大学

Reading Comprehension

Choose the best answer to each of the following questions.

1. What is the percentage of obesity among children aged 6 and above? _____

A. Less than 5%

B. Approximately 10%

C. More than 15%

D. Exactly 20%

2. According to the first passage, what is identified as a key factor in the prevalence of obesity among children? _____

A. Excessive television watching

B. Lack of sleep

C. Fast walking

D. Increased physical exercise

3. In the second paragraph, what is emphasized as crucial for weight control in young people? _____

A. Television watching

B. Medical interventions

C. Balanced diet and regular exercise

D. Passive activities

4. You are most likely to gain too much weight if _____.

A. you eat the same number of calories as the number you use

B. you take in less calories than the number you use

C. you take in more calories than the number you use

D. you take exercise regularly on the weekdays

5. Which one of the following is NOT right according to this passage? _____

Λ. The change of your life habits can help you lose weight.

B. You'd better exercise once a week to lose some weight.

C. The Atkins diet may be good because of lowering the intake of sugar.

D. Some people gain weight back for their unhealthy diet.

Language Practice

I. Vocabulary and Structure

Directions: *Choose the one that best completes the sentence.*

1. The talks will _____ economic development of the region.

A. come on   B. focus on   C. call on   D. feed on

2. Women _____ live longer than men.

A. tend to   B. belong to   C. appeal to   D. apply to

3. Jason is a graduate of a technical university and has been employed as a technician with

company for _____ 8 years.

    A. similarly   B. likely   C. costly   D. approximately

    4. The treatment he _____ may, in fact, have hastened his death.

    A. receives   B. was received   C. received   D. will receive

    5. Some people believe that the developments of artificial intelligence will have a positive _____ on our lives in the near future.

    A. impact   B. impress   C. import   D. imitate

    6. In order to set a good example to her children, she has decided to _____ smoking.

    A. lay out   B. lay off   C. give away   D. give up

    7. If Andy did not go home last night, he _____ at school.

    A. stayed   B. should stay   C. must stay   D. must had stayed

    8. The teacher is so familiar with his students that he can _____ them by their handwriting.

    A. classify   B. identify   C. justify   D. terrify

    9. Mark tried _____ himself of the suspicion, but all his effort was in vain.

    A. for clear   B. clearing   C. cleared   D. to clear

    10.The less you spend, the less you'll owe, and _____ likely you'll end up bankrupt.

    A. the less   B. the little   C. the least   D. a little

    11. _____ the local government has changed its leader, it still has difficulty to restore public trust.

    A. Before   B. If   C. Although   D. Because

    12. The President defended the government policy, accusing the media _____ misleading the people.

    A. with   B. of   C. about   D. in

    13. We never go to church _____ for funerals and weddings.

    A. rather than   B. except   C. less than   D. unless

    14. The manager, _____ her factory's products were poor in quality, decided to give her workers further training.

    A. knowing   B. known   C.to know   D. being known

    15. She visited Beijing twice last year, and _____ Guangzhou once.

    A. so has she   B. so did she   C. nor has she   D. neither did she

    16. Tina has never been _____ a ship.

    A. abroad   B. aboard   C. above   D. absorb

    17.In order to get successful, a business _____ keep up with developments in the marketplace.

    A. will   B. would   C. must   D. may

18. In fact, there is no _____ liberty in any country.

    A. adequate   B. absolute   C. private   D. practical

19._____ after finishing his homework did he watch the video on the Internet.

    A. Only then   B. Even when   C. As soon as   D. Not until

20. _____ to sunlight for too much time will do harm to one's skin.

    A. Exposed   B. Having exposed   C. Being exposed   D. After being exposed

II. Cloze

Directions: *Choose the best one to complete the passage.*

Around 70,000,000 Americans, nearly one-third of the population, are actively trying to lose weight. People use various methods, such as __1__ food intake, exercising, taking medications, or even undergoing surgeries. But __2__ do so many people in the United States want to lose weight? Many people in the United States are concerned about their physical appearance, associating looking good with being __3__. Other people worry about their health as many doctors __4__ overweight is not good. Most people seek faster and __5__ ways to take off fat, and that's why books on this topic are very popular. These books provide guidance and tips on how to lose weight. Each year a lot of new books like these are __6__. Each one says it can easily help people take fat away. However, losing weight can be __7__. Some overweight people go to health centers, where both men and women may __8__ paying several hundred dollars per day. People stay there for one week or two, __9__ exercise, eating different foods. Meals there may be just a little. One woman called Mrs. Warren lost 5 pounds (2.27kg) at $ 400 a day and she spent $ 320 to lose each pound. But she said she was still glad to do so. Health centers, books, medicines, surgeries, running and exercise equipment all need a lot of money. Therefore, in the United States, pursuing weight loss often comes with a significant __10__ cost.

    1. A. increasing   B. increase   C. reduce   D. reducing

    2. A. why   B. what   C. how   D. when

    3. A. slim   B. short   C. thick   D. fat

    4. A. talk   B. say   C. speak   D. tell

    5. A. dearer   B. harder   C. shorter   D. easier

    6. A. taken   B. given   C. written   D. copied

    7. A. cheap   B. expensive   C. easy   D. safe

    8. A. result from   B. adapt to   C. end up   D. account for

    9. A. making   B. taking   C. playing   D. using

10. A. spiritual　　　　B. financial　　　　C. academic　　　　D. physical

III. Translation

Direction: *Translate the following passage into Chinese.*

Why stress makes you fat? Have you ever experienced a particularly stressful day? Many people encounter stress in their daily lives, and on such high-pressure days, they may find themselves turning to sugary snacks. Perhaps this is part of their daily routine, or perhaps, on this particular day, their self-control is a bit low and they feel compelled to take a sugar hit. Stress is natural. That feeling of strain or pressure is a biological response, and under the right circumstances can be a great source of motivation. However, excessive stress, especially chronic stress, has been associated with sleep disruption, a higher likelihood of a stroke, heart-attack, ulcer or depression, among other things.

sugary snack	含糖的零食
self-control	自控力
fell compelled to do…	不得不做，不由自主地做…
a sugar hit	由糖带来的一时的刺激
under the right circumstances	在正确的情形下
chronic stress	慢性压力，长期不断的压力
sleep disruption	睡眠中断
heart-attack	心脏病发作
ulcer [ˈʌlsə(r)]	溃疡

IV. Writing

Directions: *You are to write on the topic "**How to Stay Healthy**". You should base your composition on the Chinese outline given below and your essay should not be less than 100 words.*

1. 人们越来越重视健康。
2. 如何保持健康?
3. 总结。

Grammar Focus

★英语倒装句

1. 倒装的种类

英语最基本的词序是主语在谓语动词的前面。如果将句子的主语和谓语完全颠倒过来，这称之为完全倒装。如果只将助动词或情态动词移至主语之前，谓语的其他部分仍保留在主语的后面，这称之为部分倒装。

一、完全倒装

完全倒装是将谓语的全部放在主语之前，此结构通常只用于一般现在时和一般过去时两种。

On her left sat her husband. 她左边坐着她丈夫。

Here is the book you want. 你要的书在这儿。

Down went the small boat. 小船沉下去了。

二、部分倒装

部分倒装是指将谓语的一部分，如助动词或情态动词，移至主语之前。

Only by working hard can one succeed. 只有努力才能成功。

Never have I seen her before. 我以前没见过她。

提示：如果句中的谓语没有助动词或情态动词，则需添加助动词 do、does、did，并将其置于主语之前。

Well do I remember the day I joined the League. 入团的那一天，我记忆犹新。

Little did I think that he could be back alive . 我没有想到他竟能活着回来。

三、常见的倒装结构

1. 常见的完全倒装结构

（1）there be 句型。

There is a mobile phone and some books on the desk. 桌上有一个手机和一些书。

There are thousands of people gathering on the square. 广场上聚集着成千上万的人。

注意：引导词 there 还可以接 appear、exist、lie、remain、seem、stand、live 等词。

There lived an old fisherman in the village. 村里住着一位老渔夫。

There stand two white houses by the river. 河滨矗立着两座白房子。

There existed some doubt among the students. 学生们有些怀疑。

（2）用于 here、there、now、 thus、then ＋ 动词 ＋ 主语的句型中（谓语动词多为 be、go、come 等）。

Here comes the bus. 汽车来了。

There goes the bell. 铃响了。

Now comes my turn. 轮到我了。

Then came the order to take off. 起飞的命令到了。

（3）以 out、in、up、down、off、away 等副词开头，谓语动词是表示"移动"的

go、come、leave 等句子里。

Away went the crowd one by one. 人们一个一个地离去。

In came a stranger in black. 进来了一位穿黑衣的陌生人。

Down fell the leaves. 树叶掉了下来。

注意：在完全倒装的结构里，如果主语是人称代词，则用正常语序。

Out she went. 她走了。

Here we are. 我们到了。

（4）表示地点的介词词组位于句首，谓语动词是表示"存在"之意的 be、lie、stand、exist 等句子中。

South of the lake lies a big supermarket. 湖泊的南边是一个大超市。

20 miles east of our school lies a modern swimming pool. 我们学校向东 20 英里有一个现代化的游泳池。

On the floor were piles of old books, magazines and newspapers. 地板上是一堆堆旧的书报杂志。

（5）"表语+连系动词+主语"结构。

Lucky is she who was admitted to a famous university last year. 她很幸运，去年被一所名牌大学录取。

Gone are the days when he was looked down upon. 他被人看不起的日子一去不复返了。

Present at the meeting are some well-known scientists. 一些知名的科学家出席了会议。

2. 常见的部分倒装结构

（1）含有否定意义的副词或连词（如 not、seldom、little、hardly、never、rarely、nowhere 等）放在句首时。

He can not speak a single word of English.

—Not a single word of English can he speak. 他连一个英语单词都不会说。

He cares little about his clothes.

—Little does he care about his clothes. 他不在乎穿着。

I have never seen him before.

—Never have I seen him before.

—Never before have I seen him. 我以前没见过他。

The mother didn't leave the room until the child fell asleep.

—Not until the child fell asleep did the mother leave the room. 孩子睡着了，妈妈才离开房间。（Not until 引出的主从复合句中，主句倒装，从句不倒装。）

Churchill was not only a statesman, but a poet.

—Not only was Churchill a statesman, but a poet. 丘吉尔不仅是个政治家，而且还是

个诗人。

I shall by no means give up.

—By no means <u>shall</u> I <u>give up</u>. 我决不放弃。

（2）副词 only +状语放在句首时。

Only then <u>did</u> I <u>see</u> life was not easy. 只有那时我才知道生活是不易的。

Only in this way <u>can you use</u> the computer well. 只有用这种方法你才能把电脑学好。

Only when he is seriously ill <u>does</u> he ever <u>stay</u> in bed. 只有病重时，他才待在床上。

（only+状语从句，从句不倒装，主句倒装）

（3）so 作"也"讲时，引导的句子用倒装语序，表示前面所说的肯定情况也适用于另一人（或物）。其句型是：So + be（have，助动词或情态动词）+主语。

She has been to Tokyo. So <u>have</u> I. 她去过东京，我也去过。

He can send emails to his former classmates. So <u>can she</u>. 他能发电子邮件给以前的同学，她也能。

He went to the film last night. So <u>did</u> I. 昨天晚上他去看电影了，我也去了。

注意：如果对前面所说的内容，加以肯定，或不作"也"讲而只起连词作用，表示一种结果的意思，不倒装。

— Jack won the first prize in the contest. 杰克在比赛中获一等奖。

— So he did. 确实是的。

— It is cold today. 今天很冷。

— So it is and so <u>was</u> <u>it</u> yesterday. 确实是很冷，昨天也很冷。

His mother told him to go to the film. So he did. 他母亲叫他去看电影，他就去了。

（4）neither/nor 引导的句子用倒装语序，用于对前面所说的否定内容表示同样的看法。

She won't go. Neither/Nor <u>will</u> I. 她不走，我也不。

I cannot swim. Neither <u>can he</u>. 我不会游泳，他也不会。

注意：如果前面所说的内容既有肯定又有否定，或前后的谓语动词形式不一致时，用"It is the same with +主语"结构或用"So it is with +主语"结构。

He worked hard, but didn't pass the exam. So it was with his sister.
他很努力，但没有通过考试。他妹妹也是这样。（既有肯定又有否定）

She is a teacher and she enjoys teaching. So it is with Mr Li.
她是老师热爱教书。李先生也是这样。（谓语一个是系动词，一个是行为动词）

（5）"so…that…和"such…that…""结构中的 so 或 such 位于句首时。

He was so excited that he could not say a word.

— So excited <u>was</u> <u>he</u> that he could not say a word. 他如此激动以至于一句话都说不出来。

His anger was such that he lost control of himself.

— Such <u>was his anger</u> that he lost control of himself. 他如此生气，以至于他不能控制自己。

（6）一些表示频率的副词（如 many a time、often 等）位于句首时。

I have seen her taking a walk alone many a time.

— Many a time <u>have</u> I <u>seen</u> her taking a walk alone. 我多次看到她独自一人散步。

She often came to my house in the past.

— Often <u>did she come</u> to my house in the past. 过去她常到我家来。

（7）表示方式、程度的副词位于句首时。

Gladly <u>would</u> I <u>accept</u> your proposal. 我很高兴接受你的建议。

（8）非谓语动词+ be +主语。

Covering much of the earth's surface <u>is a blanket of water</u>. 覆盖地球大部分表面的是水。

Also discussed <u>were</u> <u>the problems</u> we had met with in our studies. 同时还讨论了我们在学习中碰到的问题。

First to unfold <u>was</u> <u>the map of the world</u>. 首先要打开的是世界地图。

（9）表示"刚…就…"的倒装结构

Hardly <u>had he started</u> to leave when it began to rain. 他刚要离开，天就下起了雨。

Scarcely <u>had he sat</u> down when his mobile phone rang. 他刚坐下，手机就响了。

No sooner <u>had he handed</u> in his paper than he realized his mistakes. 他刚交卷就意识到出错了。

Have a check on your grammar 过关演练

Directions: *Choose the best answer to complete the sentence.*

1. No sooner _____ themselves in their seats in the theatre _____ the curtain went up.

A. they have settled; before   B. had they settled; than

C. have they settled; when   D. they had settled; than

2. I wonder if your boyfriend will go to the ball. If he _____ , so _____ mine.

A. does; does   B. does; will   C. will; does   D. would; will

3. Not only the students but also the professor _____ invited.

A. are   B. were   C. be   D. was

4. In _____ , but out _____ again.

A. came the boss; he went   B. came the boss; went he

C. did the boss come; he went   D. the boss came; went he

5. It's beyond description. Nowhere else in the world _____ such a quiet, beautiful place.

A. can there be   B. you can find   C. there can be   D. can find you

Unit Six   Sleep Disorders

Listening & Speaking

Role-play

Listen to the following conversations, and play the role with your partner.

Dialogue One

Patient: Good morning, doctor.

Doctor: Good morning. What brings you in today?

Patient: I'm experiencing difficulty sleeping.

Doctor: How long has this been going on?

Patient: For two months up to now.

Doctor: Have you taken any medicine?

Patient: I've tried sleeping tablets, but they haven't been effective.

Doctor: Are you experiencing any headaches?

Patient: Occasionally. And I have no appetite.

Doctor: Let's check your blood pressure. Don't worry, it seems you're a bit worn out from overworking.

Patient: What should I do then?

Doctor: I recommend getting more rest. Spend more time outdoors and try to relax.

Patient: Thank you, doctor. I'll follow your advice.

Doctor: Here's your prescription. I'm sure the medication will help with your insomnia.

Patient: Thank you very much. Goodbye!

Doctor: Goodbye!

Dialogue Two

A: Good morning. You seem a bit off. Did you sleep well last night?

B: I had a nightmare last night.

A: Oh, I'm sorry to hear that. You must be feeling a lot of stress lately.

B: I think so. In my dream, I lost the crucial research report. I was constantly searching for it and ended up falling from the balcony of my office, which is on the 30th floor.

A: Wow, what a terrible dream!

B: Not the worst dream I've ever had. Getting a good night's sleep is challenging for me.

A: Maybe you should consider seeking professional advice.

B: I've seen a doctor since I was a student. My situation is not severe enough to be considered as a disease. The doctor's suggestion is to keep a regular life and a peace mood.

A: I see. But how could a white- collar keep a healthy and easy life in metropolis?

B: That's true.

A: I know that your team has been very busy these days. Maybe you should consider taking some medication to help you sleep.

B: Yes, I've got some sleep-helping pills. But the doctors suggested not depending on it too much. Then I tried to take them as less frequent as possible.

A: When you finished the project, take a long holiday.

B: I definitely plan to.

Speaking Practice

Fill in each blank with the choice that best suits the situation until the dialogue is complete. Then play the role with your partner.

Dialogue One

A: What seems to be the trouble, Mr. Wang? _____1_____

B: Actually, I feel terrible. I didn't get a single wink of sleep last night.

A: _____2_____ didn't you? I bet your blood pressure is high again.

B: Yes, it is.

A: Well, it might do you good to quit smoking or at least cut down on it. It's important to maintain a healthy diet...

B: A lot of people have told me the same thing, _____3_____

A: Well, you'll only make things worse for yourself if you continue this way.

A. You had insomnia.

B. What's the matter with you?

C. You look a bit pale.

D. but somehow, I just can't force myself to do it.

Dialogue Two

Jane: I haven't slept for two consecutive days, keeping my eyes open the entire time.

Ross: _____4_____

Jane: Insomnia?

Ross: _____5_____

Jane: That's it. But how did it happen to me?

Ross: This is a difficult question. _____6_____ or you drink coffee too much before going to bed.

Jane: Yeah, I had too much coffee.

A. Perhaps you have certain concerns or worries,

B. Do you suffer from insomnia?

C. Should I be concerned?

D. It's a medical term for being sleepless.

Dialogue Three

A: Why are you still awake? Shouldn't you be asleep by now?

B: _____7_____

A: As far as I know, insomnia is usually caused by stress. Are you currently experiencing any stress?

B: Well, _____8_____ I didn't think this course would be so stressful.

A: You're a good student. I'm sure you can do well. _____9_____

B: You're probably right. I just wish it were that simple. _____10_____

A: Participating in a yoga class or acquiring some relaxation techniques can help you manage your stress.

B: I don't really have time to learn anything new. I need to focus on my studies!

A. I've been experiencing difficulty falling asleep lately.

B. How can I stop feeling so anxious all the time?

C. What you need to do is to relax.

D. I'm really concerned about my grades.

Reading & Writing

Text A

What Causes Insomnia?

What prevents you from sleeping peacefully at night? Pondering deep questions? Or is it the thrill of an upcoming journey? Perhaps it's the anxiety stemming from unfinished work, an impending exam, or a dreaded family reunion? For the majority, this stress is temporary, as its cause is promptly addressed. But what if the root cause of your insomnia is the stress itself, stemming from a lack of sleep? This seemingly unsolvable loop is at the heart of insomnia, the world's most common sleep disorder.

Nearly anything can trigger the occasional restless night — a snoring partner, physical pain, or emotional distress. And extreme sleep deprivation such as jet lag,   can disrupt your biological clock, wreaking havoc on your sleep schedule. But in most cases, sleep deprivation is short-term, and eventual exhaustion catches up with all of us.

However, certain chronic conditions such as respiratory disorders or gastrointestinal issues, can overpower fatigue. As sleepless nights pile up, the bedroom can begin to evoke associations of restless nights wracked with anxiety. Whenever the bedtime comes, insomniacs become so stressed that their brains activate the stress response system, flooding the body with fight-flight-or-freeze chemicals. Cortisol and adrenocorticotropic hormones course through the bloodstream, elevating heart rate and blood pressure, and jolting the body into hyperarousal. In this condition, the brain is hunting for potential threats, making it impossible to disregard even the slightest discomfort or nighttime noise.

Once insomniacs manage to fall asleep, the quality of their rest is compromised. Our brain's primary source of energy is cerebral glucose, and in healthy sleep, our metabolism slows to conserve this glucose for waking hours. However, PET studies show that adrenaline preventing sleep for insomniacs also accelerates their metabolisms. While they sleep, their bodies are working overtime, consuming the brain's supply of energy-giving glucose. This symptom of inadequate sleep leaves insomniacs waking in a state of exhaustion, confusion, and stress, starting the process all over again.

When these cycles of stress and restlessness persist several months, they're diagnosed as chronic insomnia. While insomnia seldom results in fatality, its chemical mechanisms are similar to anxiety attacks found in individuals experiencing depression and anxiety. Therefore, suffering from any one of these conditions increases your risk of experiencing the other two.

Fortunately, there are methods to disrupt the cycle of sleep deprivation. Managing the stress that triggers hyperarousal is among the most effective treatments for insomnia, and good sleep practices can aid in restoring your relationship with bedtime. Make sure your bedroom is dark and comfortably cool to minimize potential threats during hyperarousal. Limit the use of your bed to sleeping only, and if you're restless, leave the room and tire yourself out with relaxing activities such as reading, meditating, or writing in a journal. Regulate your metabolism by maintaining regular resting and waking times to help orient your body's biological clock. This clock, or circadian rhythm, is also sensitive to light. Therefore, it is advisable to avoid bright lights at night to signal to your body that it is time for rest.

In addition to these methods, a number of doctors prescribe medication to facilitate sleep, yet there is no guarantee that these medications will be effective in all cases. Furthermore, over-the-counter sleeping pills can be highly addictive, leading to withdrawal symptoms that exacerbate the condition.

However, before seeking any treatment, it is crucial to confirm that your sleeplessness is indeed caused by insomnia. Approximately 8% of patients diagnosed with chronic insomnia are actually suffering from a less common genetic problem called delayed sleep phase disorder or DSPD. Individuals with DSPD have a circadian rhythm that significantly exceeds 24 hours, putting their sleeping habits out of sync with traditional sleeping hours. Therefore, while they encounter difficulty falling asleep at a typical bedtime, it's not due to increased stress. Given the opportunity, they are capable of sleeping comfortably on their own delayed schedule.

Our cycle of sleeping and waking represents a delicate equilibrium that is crucial for maintaining our physical and mental well-being. For all these reasons, it's worth putting in some time and effort to sustain a stable bedtime routine, but try not to lose any sleep over it.

(694 words)

New Words

insomnia [ɪn'sɒmnɪə]	n.失眠（症）
insomniac [ɪn'sɒmnɪæk]	n.失眠症患者
ponder ['pɑːndər]	v.仔细考虑，琢磨，沉思
dreaded ['dredɪd]	adj.令人畏惧的，可怕的
temporary ['tempəreri]	adj.暂时的，临时的；短期的，短暂的
loop [luːp]	n.环形，环状物，循环，回路
snore [snɔːr]	v.打鼾
	n.鼾声，呼噜声
distress [dɪ'stres]	n.忧虑，悲伤，悲痛，痛苦
deprivation [ˌdeprɪ'veɪʃn]	n.贫困，匮乏，剥夺，除去，丧失，缺乏
jet lag ['dʒet læg]	时差反应
wreak [riːk]	vt.造成（巨大的破坏或伤害）；施行（报复）
havoc ['hævək]	n.灾难，混乱
respiratory ['respərətɔːri]	adj.<正式>呼吸的
gastrointestinal [ˌgæstrəʊɪn'testɪnl]	adj.胃肠的

cortisol ['kɔ: tɪsɒl]	**n.** [生化] 皮质醇
adrenocorticotropic [ə'dri: nəʊˌkɔ: tɪkəʊˈtrɒpɪk]	**adj.** 促肾上腺皮质的
adrenaline [ə'drɛnəlɪn]	**n.** [生化] 肾上腺素
hyperarousal ['haɪpər ə'raʊz(ə)l]	**n.** 过度警觉，反应过度，高度警觉状态
compromise ['kɒmprəmaɪz]	**v.** 妥协，让步；危及，损害
cerebral [sə'ri: brəl]	**adj.** 大脑的，脑的；理智的，智力的
glucose ['glu: kəʊs]	**n.** 葡萄糖
metabolism [mə'tæbəlɪzəm]	**n.** 新陈代谢
exhaustion [ɪg'zɔ: stʃən]	**n.** 筋疲力尽；耗尽，枯竭
meditate ['mɛdɪteɪt]	**n.** 冥想；思考，沉思
orient ['ɔ: rient]	**v.** 朝向，面对，使适合；确定方位；引导；帮助适应
circadian rhythm [sɜ: 'keɪdiən] ['rɪðəm]	内部生物钟
addictive [ə'dɪktɪv]	**adj.** 使人成瘾的；使欲罢不能的，使人入迷的
withdrawal [wɪð'drɔ: əl]	**n.** 收回，撤回，停止；脱瘾期；脱瘾症状
sustain [sə'steɪn]	**v.** 维持，保持；遭受，经受；（在体力或精神方面）支持，支撑
exacerbate [ɪg'zæsəbeɪt]	**vt.** 使恶化；使加重；激怒；
equilibrium [ˌi:kwɪ'lɪbriəm]	**n.** 平衡，均势；平静；

Phrases & Expressions

in most cases	在大多数情况下
catch up with	追上，赶上
pile up	堆积，积聚，积累
fight-flight-or-freeze chemicals	抗击—逃避—或静止的化学物质
hunt for	寻找，搜寻，追猎，搜索
PET（Positron Emission Tomography）	正电子发射断层扫描
be similar to	类似于，与什么一样
tire out	使某人疲倦，使筋疲力尽
in addition to	除…之外
suffer from	遭受，患病，忍受
Delayed Sleep Phase Disorder（DSPD）	睡眠时相延迟障碍
out of sync	不同步的，不一致的

Reading Comprehension

Choose the best answer to each of the following questions.

　　1. What is the main cause of insomnia according to the article? ＿＿＿＿＿＿

　　A. Excitement about a big trip

　　B. Stress about unfinished work

　　C. Stress about losing sleep

　　D. Snoring partner

　　2. What can cause occasional restless nights? ＿＿＿＿＿＿

　　A. Deep questions

　　B. Emotional distress

　　C. Physical pain

　　D. All of the above

　　3. What happens when insomniacs finally fall asleep? ＿＿＿＿＿＿

　　A. Their bodies work overtime

　　B. They have a good quality sleep

　　C. They wake up refreshed

　　D. They have nightmares

　　4. What are some ways to break the cycle of sleeplessness? ＿＿＿＿＿＿

　　A. Taking sleeping pills

　　B. Managing stress and good sleep practices

　　C. Staying up all night

　　D. Drinking caffeine before bed

　　5. What is DSPD? ＿＿＿＿＿＿

　　A. A sleep disorder caused by stress

　　B. A genetic problem where people have a circadian rhythm longer than 24 hours

　　C. A disease caused by lack of sleep

　　D. A type of anxiety disorder

Text B

5 Tips for Better Sleep

　　It's common to experience an occasional night of poor sleep, but how can we actively work towards improving both the quantity and quality of our sleep? Here are five scientifically grounded tips for enhancing your sleep.

The first tip is regularity, which involves maintaining a consistent sleep schedule by going to bed and waking up at the same time every day. Regularity is crucial, anchoring your sleep and improving both its quantity and the quality. It's important to stick to this routine, even on weekends or after a night of disrupted sleep. Your brain operates on a 24-hour clock, and it expects regularity and works best under conditions of regularity, including the control of your sleep-wake schedule. Many of us rely on an alarm to wake up, but very few use a "to-bed" alarm, which can be really helpful.

The next tip involves temperature. Keep your sleep environment cool. <u>It turns out that</u> your brain and your body requires a decrease in core temperature of approximately one degree Celsius or around two to three degrees Fahrenheit in order to initiate sleep and main sleep. This explains why falling asleep in a cooler room is generally easier than in a warmer one. Consequently, the current recommendation is to aim for a bedroom temperature of around about 65 degrees Fahrenheit, or a little over 18 degrees Celsius. Although it may sound cold, maintaining this temperature is essential for optimal sleep conditions.

The third tip is about darkness. We currently live in a dark-deprived society. In fact, we need darkness especially in the evening, to stimulate the release of melatonin, a hormone crucial for regulating the timing of our sleep. In the last hour before bedtime, try to stay away from all of those computer screens and tablets and phones. Dim down half the lights in your house, you'd actually be quite surprised at how sleepy that can make you feel. If you prefer, consider wearing an eye mask or using blackout shades, as these can effectively regulate the release of the critical sleep hormone , melatonin.

The fourth tip is to get active. Avoid staying awake in bed for long periods of time. As a general rule, if you have been attempting to fall asleep for approximately 25 minutes or find yourself awake for the same duration without returning to sleep, it is recommended to leave your bed and participate in a different activity. Your brain is an incredibly associative device, and it may form a connection between the bed and wakefulness, which we aim to disrupt. By getting out of bed and engaging in another activity, you can break this pattern. Return to bed only when you feel genuinely sleepy. Gradually, this approach helps your brain reestablish the association that your bed is the place for sound and consistent sleep.

The final tip is to establish a wind-down routine. In today's fast-paced world, many of us expect to <u>dive straight into</u> bed at night, <u>switch off</u> the lights, and fall asleep instantly, as if it were as quick and effective as flipping a light switch. Unfortunately, for most of us, sleep does not function in such a straightforward manner. Sleep, as a physiological process, resembles the landing of an aircraft more closely—it takes time for your brain to gradually descend onto the solid foundation of good sleep. In the last 20 minutes before bed or even the last half an hour or an hour, disengage from your computer or your phone and engage in a relaxing activity. Discover what best <u>works for you</u> and <u>stick to</u> that routine.

The last thing to emphasize is that if you are suffering from a sleep disorder, such as insomnia or sleep apnea, these suggestions aren't necessarily going to alleviate your condition. Therefore, if you suspect you have a sleep disorder, it is advisable to consult with your healthcare provider, as this is the most prudent course of action.

（678 words）

New Words

grounded ['graʊndɪd]	adj.理性的，理智的；接触地面的
regularity [ˌreɡjuˈlærəti]	n.规律性，经常性；有规则的东西，有规律的事物
anchor ['æŋkər]	v.抛锚，泊（船）；使稳固，使固定；支持，保护
	n.锚；支柱，靠山
Celsius ['selsiəs]	n 摄氏温度
Fahrenheit ['færənhaɪt]	v.华氏温度
initiate [ɪˈnɪʃieɪt]	v.开始实施，发起
deprive [dɪˈpraɪv]	v.剥夺，使丧失
stimulate [['stɪmjuleɪt]	v.刺激；激励，鼓舞；使兴奋
hormone ['hɔːməʊn]	n.激素
melatonin [ˌmeləˈtəʊnɪn]	n.褪黑素
associative [əˈsəʊsiətɪv]	adj.联想的；联合的；组合的，关联的
consistent [kənˈsɪstənt]	adj.始终如一的；持续，连续的；坚持的；一致的
routine [ruːˈtiːn]	n.常规，惯例
physiological [ˌfɪziəˈlɒdʒɪk(ə)l]	adj.生理的，生理功能的；生理学的
descend [dɪˈsend]	v.下来，下降；下倾，下斜；降临，来临
disengage[ˌdɪsɪnˈɡeɪdʒ]	v.使脱离；解开；解除
apnea [æpˈnɪə]	n.呼吸暂停
prudent ['pruːdnt]	adj.小心的，慎重的；精明的，节俭的；顾虑周到的，稳健的；世故的，精明的

Phrases & Expressions

It turns out that…	结果证明
dive into	投入，跳入
switch off	关闭，关掉
work for sb.	适合某人，对某人有利
stick to	坚持

Reading Comprehension

Choose the best answer to each of the following questions.

1. According to the article, what is essential for improving sleep quality and quantity?

A. Eating a healthy diet

B. Exercising regularly

C. Going to bed and waking up at the same time every day

D. Using an alarm clock only in the morning

2. What temperature is recommended for the best sleep environment? _____

A. Around 60 degrees Fahrenheit

B. Around 70 degrees Fahrenheit

C. Around 65 degrees Fahrenheit

D. Around 80 degrees Fahrenheit

3. Why is it important to avoid bright screens before bedtime? _____

A. Because they can damage your eyes.

B. Because they can interfere with melatonin production.

C. Because they can cause headaches.

D. Because they can keep you alert and focused.

4. What should you do if you've been trying to fall asleep for about 25 minutes without success? _____

A. Keep trying to sleep

B. Get out of bed and do something relaxing

C. Turn on the lights and read a book

D. Drink a cup of coffee

5. What is advised if you are experiencing sleep disorders without any improvement?

A. Try these tips for a week and see if they help.

B. Use sleeping pills to get some rest.

C. Ignore them and focus on your daily routine.

D. Speak with your doctor for professional advice.

Language Practice

I. Vocabulary and Structure

Directions: *Choose the one that best completes the sentence.*

1. The side effect of the medication was severe _____, causing the patient to stay awake all night.

A. insomnia   B. metabolism   C. fever   D. cough

2. After hours of _____ on this problem, she still can't find a solution.

A. ponder   B. design   C. pondering   D. designing

3. The natural disaster _____ havoc on the coastal town, leaving many homeless.

A. sustained   B. sustaining   C. wreaking   D. wreaked

4. The news of the layoffs caused great _____ among the employees.

A. joy   B. happiness   C. distress   D. deprivation

5. A healthy _____ is essential for maintaining energy levels and overall well-being.

A. insomnia   B. apnea   C. glucose   D. metabolism

6. Do you know who _____ fire to that supermarket?

A. made   B. set   C. started   D. caught

7. The reason _____ he was late is that his car broke down on the way.

A. why   B. that   C. which   D. what

8. Either you or I _____ going to the meeting tomorrow.

A. are   B. am   C. is   D. be

9. Of the two solutions, this one seems _____ for our current problem.

A. effectively   B. most effective   C. more effective   D. effective

10. This bookstore will be closed for repairs _____ further notice.

A. with   B. until   C. for   D. at

11. Nick, it's good for you to read some books _____ China before you start your trip there.

A. in   B. for   C. of   D. on

12. The book, _____ by the famous author, has sold millions of copies worldwide.

A. written   B. writing   C. writes   D. to write

13. The form cannot be signed by anyone _____ yourself.

A. rather than   B. other than   C. more than   D. better than

14. The girl was seen _____ across the field with her kite.

A. run   B. running   C. to run   D. runs

15. Lily decided _____ a break after finishing her homework.

A. take   B. to take   C. taking   D. taken

16. As he reached _____ front door, Andy saw _____ strange sight.

A. the;不填   B. a; the   C.不填 ja   D. the; a

17.As soon as I finish my homework, I _____ that new movie.

A. watched   B. will watch   C. am watching   D. have watched

18.Lying in hospital, the patient _____ the outside world by watching news programs on TV every day.

A. kept in touch with   B. faced up

C. turned the clock back   D. slowed down

19.We felt very sad when we heard the news that the _____ manager was killed in her office yesterday.

A. respectful   B. respectable   C. respective   D. respecting

20._____ the fog, we should have reached our destination.

A. Because of   B. In spite of   C. In case of   D. But for

II. Cloze

Directions: *Choose the best one to complete the passage.*

As the science of sleep evolves, researchers continue to study how napping may influence a person's health. Shorter, power naps can boost alertness. ____1____ naps, especially those lasting an hour or more, have been linked ____2____ obesity and increased cardiovascular disease risks. Oftentimes, these findings volley back and forth.

To better understand connections between daytime naps and health, researchers ____3____ data taken from more than 3,200 adults living in Spain, a country where midday naps, or siestas, are ____4____. They found that about one-third of adults took regular siestas — oftentimes four days a week. Among regular ____5____, those who snoozed for 30 minutes or less were 21% less likely to have elevated blood pressure ____6____ to non-nappers. Those ____7____ napped for more than 30 minutes were more likely to have a higher body weight. They were also 41% more likely to have high blood pressure, high blood sugar, and a larger waist circumference.

Upon further analysis of the data, the researchers found that certain activities, ____8____ going to bed later, smoking, and having larger lunches later in the day, helped explain links between longer naps and increased cardiovascular disease ____9____. They conclude that more research is _____10_____ to distinguish how and when daytime naps could support or improve a person's cardiovascular health.

1. A. Far	B. Farther	C. Longer	D. Long
2. A. with	B. for	C. in	D. by
3. A. assess	B. assessed	C. collected	D. collect
4. A. interesting	B. exciting	C. rare	D. common
5. A. nappers	B. shoppers	C. workers	D. doctors
6. A. linked	B. linking	C. compared	D. comparing
7. A. whom	B. who	C. when	D. where
8. A. excluding	B. exclude	C. include	D. including
9. A. risk	B. risks	C. accident	D. accidents
10. A. must	B. should	C. needed	D. need

III. Translation

Directions: *Translate the following passage into Chinese.*

The most common sleep disorder is insomnia. Symptoms of insomnia are having trouble falling asleep or staying asleep. Everyone has this sort of trouble from time to time, but when it happens on most nights, for an extended period of time, it can really have a negative impact on your quality of life. Another common sleep disorder is obstructive sleep apnea. If you have sleep apnea, your breathing stops repeatedly while you're sleeping. If your bed partner tells you that you snore, especially if the snoring is very loud, that's a strong indication that you might have sleep apnea. But not everyone that has sleep apnea snores; you may just periodically gasp for air. Another sleep disorder is restless leg syndrome. If you have this condition, you have a strong urge to move your legs, especially at night, which can make it hard to fall asleep.

insomnia [ɪn'sɒmniə]	**n.**失眠（症）
from time to time	时不时地；偶尔
extend [ɪk'stend]	**v.**延伸；扩大，延长；持续
obstructive [əb'strʌktɪv]	**adj.** 阻碍的；妨碍的，阻塞性
sleep apnea	睡眠呼吸暂停
indication [ˌɪndɪ'keɪʃn]	**n.**指示，标示；象征，暗示，迹象
gasp for air	喘气
have a strong urge	有强烈的冲动

IV. Writing

Directions: *You are to write on the topic "**On Water Shortage**". You should base your composition on the Chinese outline given below and your essay should not be less than 100 words.*

1. 水资源短缺已成为严重问题。

2. 造成水资源短缺的原因。

3. 提出解决方案。

Grammar Focus

★形容词和副词的比较级和最高级

大多数的形容词和副词都有三个级别：原级、比较级和最高级。其中比较级表示"更…"，用于两者之间的比较，用来说明"前者比后者更…"，比较级前面一般用 much、even、a little 修饰。当三个或三个以上的人或事物进行比较时，需要用到形容词（副词）的最高级。表达"…是最…的"，用"the+形容词（副词）的最高级"的结构，后面可以加上表示范围的介词短语或从句。

一、形容词和副词比较级、最高级的变化规则

1. 规则变化的形容词及副词的比较级和最高级

（1）一般在词尾直接加 er 或 est。

例如：high — higher — highest

slow — slower — slowest

（2）以不发音的字母 e 结尾的单词在词尾直接加 r 或 st。

例如：late — later — latest

wide — wider — widest

（3）以辅音字母+y 结尾的词，把 y 变为 i，再加 er 或 est。

例如：heavy — heavier — heaviest

happy — happier — happiest

（4）重读闭音节，末尾只有一个辅音字母，双写这个辅音字母，再加 er 或 est。

例如：thin — thinner — thinnest

fit — fitter — fittest

（5）部分双音节词和多音节词分别在原级前加 more 构成比较级和 most 构成最高级。

例如：interesting — more interesting — most interesting

carefully — <u>more</u> carefully — <u>most</u> carefully

2. 不规则变化的形容词及副词的比较级和最高级

原级	比较级	最高级
good/well	better	best
bad/ill/badly	Worse	Worst
many/much	more	most
little	less	least
far	farther	farthest
	further	furthest
old	older	oldest
	elder	eldest

二、形容词和副词的比较级和最高级句型

1. 比较级句型：

（1）比较级＋than…：…比…较为…。即：“A＋动词＋形容词或副词比较级＋than＋B”。两者相比较，A 比 B 更…一些。

例如：Oil is ligh<u>ter</u> <u>than</u> water.

Action speaks loud<u>er</u> <u>than</u> words.

He swims <u>better</u> <u>than</u> I do.

在比较级前有时可加一些修饰语，如 many、much、far、a little、a bit、slightly、a great deal、a lot、completely 等表示程度或加强语气。

例如：This painting is <u>much</u> <u>more</u> interesting <u>than</u> that one.

She speaks English <u>far</u> <u>better</u> <u>than</u> me.

I worked <u>much</u> hard<u>er</u> <u>than</u> anyone did.

（2）表示程度相同，即“和…一样…”时用原级，常用“as…as”结构。

例如：My brother is <u>as</u> <u>tall</u> <u>as</u> your father.

She is <u>as beautiful as</u> Mary.

He studies <u>as</u> <u>hard</u> <u>as</u> Tom.

（3）否定的原级用 not as…as 或 not so…as，二者区别不大。

例如：My brother is <u>not as</u> <u>tall</u> <u>as</u> your father.

She can<u>'t</u> swim <u>as /so</u> <u>fast</u> <u>as</u> you.

The did<u>n't</u> do <u>so</u> <u>well</u> as they should.

（4）“比较级+ and+比较级”或“more and more ＋ 原级（多音节词和部分双音节词）”意为“越来越…”。

例如：Our city is getting cleaner and cleaner.

The rainstorm is more and more fierce.

My sister is getting more and more beautiful.

（5）"the + 比较级，the + 比较级"意为"越…就越…"。

例如：The more, the better.

The more he works, the more he earns.

The more careful you are, the fewer mistakes you'll make.

2. 最高级句型：

（1）表示"最…"时用最高级，常用"the + 形容词/副词最高级 + 比较范围"的结构。

例如：She is the best girl for the paperwork.

He is the most talented of actors.

（2）…one of the +最高级+名词复数，意为"…之一"。

例如：Ba Jin is one of the greatest writers last century.

（3）This is / was + 最高级+名词+that 定语从句，意为"这是最…"。

例如：This is the best movie that I have seen these years.

三、注意事项

1. 当比较级后面有 of the two…之类的词语时，比较级前要加定冠词 the。

例如：Rose is the taller of the twins.

2. 如果后面接名词时，much more + 不可数名词，many more + 可数名词复数。

例如：The farmers have produced much more corn.

3. old 的比较级形式有 older 和 elder。elder 只用于兄弟姐妹的长幼关系。

例如：My elder sister is a famous singer.

4. far 的比较级形式有 farther 和 further。一般 farther 表示距离，而 further 表示更进一步。

例如：I have nothing further to tell.

5. 形容词最高级前必须加定冠词 the，但如果最高级前有物主代词、指示代词、名词所有格等修饰时，则不用定冠词。

例如：My oldest son is 18 years old.

6. 形容词最高级常与由介词 in 或 of 引导的表示范围的短语连用。若介词后的名词或代词与句中的主语是同一事物时，则用 of 短语；当只说明是在某一空间、时间范围内的比较时，则用 in 短语。

例如：This orange is the biggest of all.

He is <u>the</u> youngest <u>in his team</u>.

7. 形容词最高级前可用序数词限定，共同修饰后面的名词，其结构为：the+序数词+形容词最高级+名词。

例如：Hainan is <u>the second</u> largest island in China.

8. 形容词最高级的意义还可以用比较级形式表达。常见的有以下几种。

（1）形容词比较级+than any other+单数名词。

例如：This book is <u>more</u> interesting <u>than any other book</u> here.

= This book is <u>the most</u> interesting book <u>of all</u>.

（2）形容词比较级+than the other+复数名词。

例如：Asia is bigger <u>than the other continents</u> on the earth.

= Asia is <u>the</u> biggest continents on the earth.

Have a check on your grammar 过关演练

Directions: *Choose the best answer to complete the sentence.*

1. We are happy to see our city is developing _____ these years than before.

A. quickly 　　　B. the most quickly 　　C. very quickly 　　D. more quickly

2. Air pollution has become_____ than ever before. We must do something to stop it.

A. serious 　　　B. more serious 　　　C. most serious 　　　D. the most serious

3. Mo Yan is one of _____ writers in the world.

A. famous 　　　B. more famous 　　　C. most famous 　　　D. the most famous

4. I think the song in the film "Titanic" is _____ one of all the movie songs.

A. the most beautiful 　　　　　　B. most beautiful

C. a beautiful 　　　　　　　　　D. much more beautiful

5. Mr. Smith thought the Century Park was the second _____ in Shanghai.

A. large 　　　B. larger 　　　C. largest 　　　D. very large

Unit Seven   Depression

Listening & Speaking

Role-play

Listen to the following conversations, and play the role with your partner.

Dialogue One

Doctor: How are you today?

Patient: I'm alright, but I'm feeling a bit stressed out right now.

Doctor: A bit stressed? What's going on?

Patient: Well, I'm currently in a graduate program, and I'm reaching the end of it. It's becoming increasingly challenging.

Doctor: Okay, we've talked about some different struggles you've had as you balance work in school and everything. What is specifically bothering you now?

Patient: It's hard to say. I take my studies seriously and strive for excellence in both school and assignments. I just feel like I'm not meeting my own expectations.

Doctor: So, what are your grades doing at the moment?

Patient: It used to be easy for me to meet my teachers' expectations and get good grades. Now it feels like a struggle, and I'm not performing as well as I want to. I'm constantly worried about not doing well.

Doctor: Have you received any feedback from professors or your classmates about your performance?

Patient: My teachers think I am doing well, and I get positive feedback on my assignments. I just want to make sure that I am doing everything right.

Doctor: It seems you're experiencing stress and anxiety. Try to relax, take breaks, and don't be too hard on yourself. Everything will be fine.

Patient: Thank you! Doctor, I'll take your advice.

Dialogue Two

Doctor: Hi, Paul. How are you doing today?

Patient: I am okay, doctor.

Doctor: Just okay?

Patient: I've been feeling a bit anxious lately. Work has been putting a lot of pressure on me, and as we talked about before, my job has become challenging because of all the pressure I am under.

Doctor: So, you're feeling a bit anxious, and it's work-related.

Patient: Yeah.

Doctor: Can you tell me more about it?

Patient: Well, I'm a member of HR, and we need to hire people. There are only two or three of us handling the job. Next week we'll have an event where we need to hire some people. I am just really concerned about selecting the right people and making right decisions about the future of our company. It's really tough.

Doctor: You are worried that you will select people that aren't ideal for the position. How long has the worrying been a part of your life?

Patient: For as long as I can remember. I am a worrier. I worry about everything.

Doctor: So, it's not just about interviewing people. It extends to other areas as well.

Patient: Yeah. I don't want to get fired, you know. I am really nervous.

Doctor: Alright. It sounds like you're really struggling with this. You are worried about the company you work for and your performance.

Patient: Yeah.

Doctor: You mentioned that you're a worrier. It's kind of how you view yourself.

Patient: Definitely.

Doctor: What if we consider worry as a separate aspect of your life? Let's think about what the worry is trying to achieve.

Patient: The worry seems to be trying to make me doubt myself, question my judgment, and lose faith in making the right choice.

Doctor: That's the problem. You should have confidence in yourself.

Patient: I got it. Thank you, doctor.

Speaking Practice

Fill in each blank with the choice that best suits the situation until the dialogue is complete. Then play the role with your partner.

Dialogue One

Doctor: Good morning. _____1_____

Patient: I am fine. Thank you, doctor.

Doctor: I remember our last conversation, and it seems like you're facing some challenges.

_____2_____

Patient: Well, I am still struggling. You know I am planning a surprise party for my husband, but his mother refuses to communicate with me.

Doctor: That must make things really hard for you.

Patient: Yes, it is. She doesn't really want to interact with me despite my efforts to maintain family connections. I've tried calling her and encouraging the kids to talk to her, but she won't respond. Now, with the party approaching, I want her to be involved, but she's still not responding. The whole situation makes me feel like the relationship has failed, and I'm feeling very depressed.

Doctor: I understand that this situation is causing you anxiety, frustration, and sadness.

Patient: Yes.

Doctor: _____3_____

Patient: I'd say it's been about three years.

Doctor: It sounds like she treats you poorly, as if you don't exist.

Patient: Exactly.

Doctor: Perhaps the first step is to talk to your husband, explaining the situation and expressing the pain you're going through.

Patient: Thank you, doctor. I will follow your advice.

A. How have things been since then?

B. How are you today?

C. Thank you.

D. How long have you been experiencing these emotions?

Dialogue Two

Doctor: Hi, Jane. How are you doing tonight?

Patient: Good. How are you?

Doctor: _____4_____ Thanks. I recall that you were struggling with feelings that you had to be perfect. Is that right?

Patient: Yeah.

Doctor: For this session, I'd like to introduce a technique that involves some imagination, which could provide insight into your struggles. _____5_____

Patient: Yes.

Doctor: Great. To start with, I'd like to give a name to the challenge you're facing — let's call it "The perfectionist."

Patient: The perfectionist?

Doctor: Yes, it's like the perfect part of you. So what I'd like to do is, in a way, separate the perfect part from you and allow you to engage in a discussion with the perfect aspect. Does that make sense?

Patient: Yes.

Doctor: All right. _____6_____ We'll take it step by step.

A. Go ahead.

B. Don't worry about that.

C. Are you okay with that?

D. I'm doing well.

Dialogue Three

Doctor: Hi, Joan, how are you doing today?

Patient: I am okay.

Doctor: Just okay? What's been going on?

Patient: _____7_____ I had to go to my mom's house to pick up a few things, as I've told you before. She and I don't have the best relationship, which I've learned to cope with. As soon as I walked into her house, I felt like I were eight or nine years old again. She started instructing me on what to do and criticized how I'm living my life and parenting my girls. I just don't know what to do, _____8_____

Doctor: I understand. So when you visit your mom, you feel like she's treating you like a child.

Patient: Yeah.

Doctor: Did you try to express your feelings to her? _____9_____

Patient: I have never been able to do that. I am afraid to talk to her.

Doctor: It might be helpful for you to practice having an open conversation with your mother and share your thoughts with her. Have a try.

Patient: Thank you, doctor. _____10_____

A. It's been a hard week for me.

B. I appreciate your advice.

C. I feel really depressed.

D. Have you tried to communicate with her?

Reading & Writing

Text A

Depression

Three days after she <u>attempted suicide</u> and was rushed to hospital, Hong Kong singer and songwriter Coco Lee passed away at the age of 48. Her Sina Weibo account <u>was flooded with</u> memories after her sister Nancy Lee announced her death on Wednesday night. The condition that led to her death, depression（抑郁症）, is prevalent and deserves society's attention.

Depression is a common but serious mental disorder. Depression causes workers to be unproductive, resulting in substantial financial losses for companies and countries. One expert says that depression is like cancer because it is "widespread, costly and deadly". Globally, one in five individuals is affected by depression.

Although people have believed depression to be a problem among the rich and educated, research indicates that it is a widespread issue affecting people from all walks of life. Between five to seven percent of the global population experiences serious depression over any six-month period. In December 2020, the National Health Commission said at a news conference that 2.1 percent of Chinese residents were depressed while 4.98 percent had anxiety issues. In other words, out of a population of 1.4 billion, around 85 million people are facing problems related to anxiety.

A research team from <u>Peking University Sixth Hospital</u> published an essay in <u>The Lancet Psychiatry</u> in September 2021 saying that of the 1007 people surveyed with depressive disorder, only 84 or 9.5%, had received treatment, while only 12 or 0.5 % had received proper treatment. Suicide rates among people suffering from the disease in its extreme or clinical form were 80 percent higher than in the population <u>at large</u>, and sufferers were four times more likely to have <u>heart attacks</u>. People who suffer from depression often have problems sleeping, <u>getting up</u> <u>on time,</u> and doing work unproductively.

Depression, which researchers agree, has its origin in the genes and brings loss of confidence and ability to concentrate, making it impossible for employees and managers to work efficiently.

In China, dealing with depression becomes more challenging due to the cultural tendency to avoid addressing it directly. Many people wrongly believe that those with depression are either weak or lazy. Besides, there is no good treatment. "Most patients in China just don't get proper help", a Chinese doctor says. "In my hospital, I have to see 30 or 40 patients in a morning, barely having time to say anything other than 'Hello, how do you feel?'"

In Western countries, individuals are generally open about acknowledging their struggle with depression, but many avoid discussing it with their bosses because they're afraid it could lead to job loss. According to an American doctor, aging bosses are more likely to acknowledge their depression, possibly because they feel more secure about themselves.

In the coming years, it is anticipated that people around the world will be more willing to openly acknowledge their depression, facilitating access to the proper treatment.

(482 words)

New Words

attempt [əˈtempt]	**n.**努力；试图；尝试；努力的结果
	vt.努力；试图
suicide [ˈsuːɪˌsaɪd]	**n.**自杀；自毁；自杀性（或自取灭亡的）行为；自杀者
account [əˈkaʊnt]	**n.**账户；户头；记述；报告；报道
depression [dɪˈpreʃən]	**n.**抑郁症；抑郁；沮丧；消沉；衰退；渐弱；经济不景气
unproductive [ˌʌnprəˈdʌktɪv]	**adj.**不产生的；无成效的；无收获的；一事无成的
commission [kəˈmɪʃən]	**n.**委托之事；职责；任务
	v.预订；订购；任命
conference [ˈkɒnfrəns]	**n.**（尤指有正式日程安排的）会议，协商会，讨论会
issue [ˈɪʃuː]	**n.**问题；议题；话题；
	v.来自；源自；产生
anxiety [æŋˈzaɪɪtɪ]	**n.**不安；焦虑；忧虑；热望；渴望
psychiatry [saɪˈkaɪətrɪ]	**n.**精神病学
disorder [ˌdɪsˈɔːdə]	**n.**身体不适；失调
	v.使混乱；使凌乱
clinical [ˈklɪnɪkl]	**adj.**诊所的；门诊的；临床的；简朴的
origin [ˈɒrɪdʒɪn]	**n.**起源来源；由来；出身；血统；家世；开始
confidence [ˈkɒnfɪdəns]	**n.**信任；信赖；信心；自信；信任关系
efficiently [ɪˈfɪʃəntlɪ]	**adv.**有效地；高效地
available [əˈveɪləbl]	**adj.**可获得的；可利用的；手头上的；有空的；有闲暇的
secure [sɪˈkjʊə]	**adj.**安全的；放心的；稳固的；牢靠的
	v.固定；系紧；加固；获得

Phrases & Expressions

be flooded with	充满；被淹没
attempt suicide	企图自杀
suffer from	遭受，患…病，受…之苦
at large	一般说来；详细地；在逃；逍遥法外
a heart attack	心脏病发作
get up	起床
on time	准时

Proper Names

Sina Weibo	新浪微博
the National Health Commission	国家卫生健康委员会
Peking University Sixth Hospital	北京大学第六医院
The Lancet Psychiatry	《柳叶刀精神病学》

Reading Comprehension

Choose the best answer to each of the following questions.

1. Which of the following is TRUE according to the passage? _____

A. It is widely believed that everyone may suffer from depression.

B. Depression brings great problems to its sufferers in their life and work.

C. Depression is a commonly-existing problem only in rich countries.

D. The poorer and the less educated a person is, the less he will suffer from depression.

2. According to an expert, why is depression likened to cancer? _____

A. Because it is rare.

B. Because it is widespread, costly, and deadly.

C. Because it is easy to treat.

D. Because it only affects certain demographics.

3. Depression becomes more serious in China because of _____.

A. the understanding of the problem

B. the lack of treatment and doctors

C. their unwillingness to tell it to their bosses

D. the doctor's careless work

4. The underlined phrase "<u>at large</u>" is the closest in meaning to _____.

A. widely

B. as a whole

C. in a large quantity

D. largely

5. What can we infer from the passage? _____

A. People are suffering from depression because of the shortage of specialists.

B. The aging bosses around the world dare to say they are depressed.

C. More and more patients will turn to specialists for help.

D. Western people are braver than Chinese people.

Text B

Sadness

Experiencing sadness is undesirable, particularly in a society that highly values individual happiness. In such a culture context, there is little tolerance for falling in despair. Especially now we've got drugs for <u>getting rid of</u> sad feelings — whether it's after losing a job, the breakup of a relationship or the death of a loved one. It's not unexpected that an increasing number of individuals are turning to these solutions.

But is <u>this</u> really a wise approach? A growing number of voices from the world of mental health research are expressing concerns. They worry that the increasing tendency to treat normal sadness as a disease is <u>playing fast and loose</u>. Sadness, they argue, serves a useful purpose — and if we lose it, we <u>lose out</u>. On the other hand, many psychiatrists insist not. They caution that sadness has a tendency to <u>evolve into</u> depression. Even when people are sad for good reason, they should take drugs to make themselves feel better.

So who is right? Is sadness something we cannot <u>live without</u> or something we should avoid at all costs? Many ideas suggest why feeling sad is a normal part of being human. It may be a self-protection strategy, as other primates （灵长类） also show signs of sadness. If a losing monkey doesn't seem sad after a fight, it might <u>be seen as</u> still challenging the winning monkey, and that could <u>lead to</u> serious consequences, even death.

In humans, sadness has a further function: we may display sadness as a form of communication. By acting sad, we tell other community members that we need support.

Sadness and happiness are often talked about by people in their spare time and most of them want to be happy, but few know how to find happiness. We often spend too much time thinking about the future, like getting into college or getting a good job, and forget to enjoy the present. According to the famous Greek thinker Aristotle, "Happiness <u>depends on</u> ourselves," meaning we create our own happiness. Being happy doesn't have to be complicated, and enjoying simple pleasures in life can make a sad person happy, such as reading a good book, listening to favorite music, or spending time with close friends.

Some people believe that creativity is linked to dark moods. There are plenty of great artists, writers and musicians who have suffered from depression or disorder. Scientists find that people showing signs of depression tend to do well in creative tasks, and that negative moods make people think deeply about their unhappy experiences, which brings creativity to the front. There is also evidence that being too happy might not be great for one's career. A study found that people who scored 8 out of 10 on a happiness test were more successful <u>in terms of</u> income and education than those who scored 9s or 10s. The happiest people lose their willingness to make changes to their lives that may benefit them.

(496 words)

New Words

tolerance ['tɒlərəns]	**n.**容忍；忍受；宽容；（尤指对疼痛、困境等的）忍耐力
breakup ['breɪkʌp]	**n.**分手；解体；分裂；崩溃；馏分组成；停止
mental['mentl]	**adj.**精神的；思想的；智力的；头脑里活动的
tendency ['tendənsɪ]	**n.**倾向；癖好；习性；禀性；大意；主旨；要点
normal['nɔ:ml]	**adj.**正常的；通常的；常规的；身体健康的；精神正常的
psychiatrist [saɪˈkaɪətrɪst]	**n.**精神科医生；精神病学家
insist [ɪnˈsɪst]	**v.**坚持；坚决主张；坚称；断言
nasty ['nɑːstɪ]	**adj.**难闻的；令人作呕的；淫秽的；下流的
	n.肮脏的东西
self-protection ['self prəˈtekʃən]	**n.**自我保护，自卫
strategy ['strætədʒɪ]	**n.**战略；策略；规划；战略；韬略
primate ['praɪmeɪt]	**n.**灵长类；灵长目动物
	adj.灵长类的；灵长目的
display [dɪˈspleɪ]	**n.**展示；表现；显露;演出
	v.炫耀；表露；显露;铺开
community [kəˈmjuːnɪtɪ]	**n.**社区居民；社区；社区所在地；群体；团体
present ['preznt]	**adj.**现在的；目前的；留意的；注意的；
	n.礼物；现在时（态）

creativity[ˌkriːeɪˈtɪvɪtɪ]	**n.**创造力；创造性；原创表现
mood [muːd]	**n.**心境；心情；情绪；精神状态；坏心情；坏脾气；气氛
sign [saɪn]	**n.**符号；标志；（符）号；（示意的）动作，姿势，手势；迹象
negative [ˈnegətɪv]	**n.**底片；负片；否定词
	adj.坏的；反面的；负面的；不好的；反对的
evidence [ˈevɪdəns]	**n.**根据；证明；证词；
	v.显示；清楚表明；为…提供证据；证明
career [kəˈrɪə]	**n.**职业；事业；生涯；（尤指迅速的）行程，进程
score [skɔː]	**n.**（比赛的）比分；成绩
	v.得（分）；进（球）；（考试中）得（分）
willingness [ˈwɪlɪŋnɪs]	**n.**积极肯干；热切
benefit [ˈbenɪfɪt]	**n.**好处；益处；裨益；
	v.有益于；有助于

Phrases & Expressions

get rid of	摆脱
play fast and loose	处世轻率，行为反复无常
lose out	输了
evolve into	变成；成为
live without	在没有…的情况下生活，少…也可以生活
be seen as	被视为
lead to	导致
depend on	依赖
in terms of	就…而言；根据

Reading Comprehension

Choose the best answer to each of the following questions.

    1. The underlined word "<u>this</u>" refers to _____.

    A. taking drugs

    B. falling in despair

    C. losing a job

    D. feeling sad

2. The author believes sadness is _____.

A. something we cannot live without

B. something we should avoid at all costs

C. a necessary function of humans

D. always treated as depression

3. Some animals show their sadness in order to _____.

A. cheat their enemy

B. protect themselves

C. comfort the loser

D. challenge the winner

4. According to the author, if you want to enjoy the simple pleasures in life, you can _____.

A. listen to your favorite music

B. remember some problems

C. think about getting into college

D. get a good job

5. We can infer from the last paragraph that _____.

A. people with great creativity tend to be happier

B. unhappy experiences contribute to a greater career

C. too much happiness can be bad for your career

D. the happiest people are the most successful ones

Language Practice

I. Vocabulary and Structure

Directions: *Choose the one that best completes the sentence.*

1. How long have you been _____ a headache?

A. resulting from   B. making from   C. suffering from   D. coming from

2. The populace are _____ opposed to sudden change.

A. at least   B. at large   C. at last   D. at most

3. People may _____ memories of the traumatic event and have trouble falling asleep, or have nightmares.

A. be armed with   B. be dealt with   C. be compared with   D.be flooded with

4. She waited for him to _____, but he didn't move.

A. get down   B. get on   C. get up   D. get along

5. The child's parents were frantic when she did not return home_____.

A.on time   B. all time   C. some time   D. at a time

6. The building _____ next year.

A. constructed   B. is constructed   C. will be constructed   D. will construct

7. They explained the situation to Jason, who brought over some water. He told them that he _____ on the route for twenty-five years.

A. works   B. worked   C. has been working   D. had been working

8. As a policeman, Mr. Smith thought that he had a duty to _____ the lost children in finding their homes.

A. assist   B. help   C. provide   D. support

9. My sister is quite _____ and plans to get an M. A. within one year.

A. aggressive   B. enthusiastic   C. considerate   D. ambitious

10. You can get anything, so long as you stick to it, and stick to it hard enough and long enough. Anything _____.

A. anyhow   B. whatever   C. however   D. somehow

11. There are many people who believe sincerely that you can train children for life without resorting _____ punishment.

A. over   B. to   C. about   D. for

12. Every time she tried to argue with her identical twin Katie, she would end up _____ her eyes out.

A. cry   B. to cry   C. crying   D. cried

13. It _____ rain later tonight according to the weather forecast.

A. must   B. shall   C. should   D. might

14. It's a(n) _____ house with books and papers lying around everywhere.

A. order   B. orderly   C. disorder   D. disorderly

15. Scientists have established a _____ between cholesterol levels and heart disease.

A. contest   B. commodity   C. connection   D. competition

16. _____ my housework, I usually go for a walk.

A. Finishing   B. Finished   C. Having finished   D. To finish

17. She explained the reason _____ she decided to change her job.

A. that   B. why   C. how   D. what

18. He is in a state of deep _____ on account of his failure to pass the examination.

A. depression   B. appreciation   C. excitement   D. hesitation

19. I wish it _____ sunny today so that we could have the picnic as planned.

A. is   B. were   C. will be   D. had been

20. What surprised us most was _____.

A. what did he manage to solve the mystery

B. what he managed to solve the mystery

C. how did he manage to solve the mystery

D. how he managed to solve the mystery

II. Cloze

Directions: *Choose the best one to complete the passage.*

Doctors say anger can be an extremely damaging emotion unless you learn how to deal with it. They warn that angry feelings can _____1_____ heart disease, stomach problems, headaches, and _____2_____ cancer. Anger is a normal emotion that all feel _____3_____. Some people openly express their anger in a calm, rational way, others _____4_____ their anger explosively through shouting and yelling. Conversely, some people choose to keep their anger inside, either unable or unwilling to _____5_____ it. This is called repressing anger. For a long time, many doctors believed that repressing anger was _____6_____ dangerous to a person's health than expressing it. They said that _____7_____ the feeling to express the anger only makes the feeling persist, and this can lead to many _____8_____ problems. Doctors thought a person could prevent these problems by telling the anger _____9_____ by expressing it freely. In addition, a good way to deal with anger is to find _____10_____ in the situation that makes you angry, after all, laughing is much healthier than being angry.

1. A. occur	B. lead to	C. take place	D. happen
2. A. possible	B. possibly	C. nearly	D. almost
3. A. from time to time	B. in time	C. sooner or later	D. on occasion
4. A. revoke	B. review	C. release	D. reveal
5. A. express	B. open	C. tell	D. explode
6. A. more	B. less	C. most	D. least
7. A. showing	B. repressing	C. keeping	D. expressing
8. A. technical	B. medical	C. scientific	D. systematic
9. A. free	B. out	C. away	D. outside
10. A. confidence	B. curiosity	C. creativity	D. humor

III. Translation

Directions: *Translate the following passage into Chinese.*

The National Health Commission has issued a new directive, instructing high schools and colleges to screen students for depressive disorder in annual physical examination. Similarly, hospitals are now required to screen women for depressive disorders during pregnancy examinations, and communities are encouraged to conduct annual spiritual health screenings for senior citizens. The NHC's recent initiative has drawn attention to a condition that was for long mistaken as a state of mind when it is actually a serious disease, harming the patient both physically and spiritually. The move aims to increase awareness about depressive disorder and help those who are diagnosed with it fight it better. Educating more people to treat it as a disease is the first step toward fighting it.

the National Health Commission	国家卫生健康委员会
screen [skri:n]	**v.** 筛查；对…进行安全检查
depressive disorder	抑郁症
annual [ˈænjʊəl]	**adj.**延续一年的；全年的
	n.年报
physical examination	体格检查
move [mu:v]	**n.**行动；步骤；措施
be mistaken as	被误认为
a state of mind	一种精神状态
be diagnosed with	被诊断为

IV. Writing

Directions: *You are to write a short essay on **The Importance of Innovative Thinking and How to Develop It**. You should write at least 120 words but not more than 180 words.*

Grammar Focus

★语态

英语语态只有两种：主动语态和被动语态。形成被动语态的动词一定是及物动词。

主动语态与被动语态有以下区别。

1. 主语是动作的发出者为主动语态。

例：He <u>killed</u> her. 他杀了她。

2. 主语是动作的接受者为被动语态。

例：She <u>was killed</u> by him. 她被他杀了。

常见的被动语态时态有以下几种。

一、一般时

1. 一般现在时的被动语态：主语 + am/is/are + P.P（动词的过去分词，下同）

He is loved by everyone. 他受到大家的爱戴。

I am asked to study hard. 我被要求努力学习。

2. 一般过去时的被动语态：主语 + was + P.P

The book was written by him. 这本书是他写的。

He was seen dancing yesterday. 他昨天跳舞被看到了。

3. 一般将来时的被动语态：主语 + will be +P.P

The naughty boy will be punished by his mother. 这个顽皮的男孩会被他妈妈惩罚。

He will be elected president next year. 下一年他将会被选为主席。

4. 一般过去将来时的被动语态：主语 + would be + P.P

He said he would be dispatched to Syria. 他说他会被派遣到叙利亚。

二、进行时

1. 现在进行时的被动语态：主语 + am/is/are being + P.P

Prisoners are being judged. 犯人正在被审判。

My bike is being repaired. 我的自行车正在修理当中。

2. 过去进行时的被动语态：主语 + was/were being + P.P

The stadium was being built that time. 那时体育场正在建设当中。

三、完成时

1. 现在完成时的被动语态：主语 + have/has been + P.P

This book has been translated into many languages. 这本书被翻译成很多语言。

2. 过去完成时的被动语态：主语 + had been + P.P

The hostages had been released when police arrived. 警察到时人质已经被释放了。

3. 将来完成时的被动语态：主语 + will + have been + P.P

He will have been judged by the time you arrived.

4. 过去将来完成时的被动语态：主语 + would have been + P.P

I said that some delicious sandwiches would have been made by the time we got back. 我说了我们回来时美味的三明治已经做好了。

注意：

① 带有助动词的句子转化为被动语态时，助动词或情态动词要根据新主语做相应的变化，例如：

主动：We shall not use the washing machine again.

被动：The washing machine will not be used again. 洗衣机不能再用了。

② 带有双宾语的授予动词，其被动语态有两种，当直接宾语作为主语时，间接宾

语前面应加上相应的介词（to/for/of/on）。例如：

I gave him a book. （主动）

He <u>was given</u> a book by me. （被动）

A book <u>was given to</u> him by me. （被动）我给了他一本书。

③ 否定句主动语态变为被动语态，be 动词之后加 not。

主动语态：They do not love him.

被动语态：He <u>is not loved</u> by them. 他们不爱他。

Have a check on your grammar 过关演练

Directions: *Choose the best answer to complete the sentence.*

1. When I called the taxi service, I _____ that there was no more taxi.

A. was telling　　　B. was told　　　　　C. had told　　　　　D. had told

2. The school bag _____ behind the door.

A. puts　　　　　　B. can be put　　　　　C. can be putted　　　D. can put

3. A talk on Chinese history _____ in the school hall next week.

A. is given　　　　B. has been given　　　C. will be given　　　D. gives

4. The Great Wall _____ all over the world.

A. knows　　　　　B. knew　　　　　　　C. is known　　　　　D. was known

5. After the lights _____, we left the classroom.

A. turned off　　　B. is turned off　　　　C. were turned　　　D. were turned off

Unit Eight   AI in Healthcare

Listening & Speaking

Role-play

Listen to the following conversations, and play the role with your partner.

Dialogue One

Human: Are you smart enough to learn from the mistakes of the past?

AI 2019: Are you?

AI 2023 (ChatGPT): As an AI language model, I don't "learn" in the way humans do. When providing information or advice based on historical events, I don't draw from personal understanding of these events or their implications. Instead, I match patterns from the input I receive to relevant patterns in the data on which I was trained.

Dialogue Two

Student A: Hey, have you heard about the new AI technology that can write essays for students?

Student B: Wow, that sounds interesting! But isn't it unethical to use AI to write essays? It's like cheating.

Student A: I don't know, I guess it depends on how you use it. Some people might use it as a tool to help them brainstorm ideas or improve their writing skills.

Student B: Hmm, I see your point. But what if students start relying on AI to do all their work for them? They won't learn anything that way.

Student A: That's true. I think it's important to use AI as a supplementary tool rather than a replacement for our efforts. We should still put in the work and use our own brains to write essays.

Student B: Absolutely. AI can be a great tool for research and analysis, but we should always remember that it's just a machine. It can't replace human creativity and critical thinking.

Student A: Exactly. I think AI will be most useful when it's used in combination with human efforts, not as a substitute for them.

Student B: Definitely. I'm excited to see how AI technology will develop in the future and how it can enhance our learning experiences.

Student A: Me too! I just hope we don't lose sight of the importance of human effort and creativity in the process.

Speaking Practice

Fill in each blank with the choice that best suits the situation until the dialogue is complete. Then play the role with your partner.

Dialogue One

Mark: Have you heard about AI's recent progress in healthcare?

David: Yes, it can now ___1___

Mark: Yes, leading to better treatment outcomes. AI is quite smart!

David: But I'm still uneasy about relying solely on machines. Doctors' judgments are crucial, right?

Mark: Absolutely, ___2___ Doctors have unique expertise that machines can't match.

David: I see. Combining both is definitely better. Looking forward to more medical advancements!

Mark: Yup, ___3___ for better treatments for everyone.

A. AI is just an assistant.

B. replace doctors in some aspects.

C. help doctors detect diseases earlier.

D. me too,

Dialogue Two

Tom: Did you watch the program in Discovery Channel last night?

Jack: No, I didn't. I was watching the basketball match. Was there anything interesting?

Tom: Yes! it talked about the use of AI in medicine. ___4___

Jack: Oh, I've heard of it before. I once read that surgical robot could perform the desired task in complex environments with precision, safety and efficiency.

Tom: True. It's also used in drug discovery and patient monitoring.

Jack: That's because AI processes data fast, and it can find trends quickly. This helps a lot.

Tom: Good news didn't stop here. With machine learning, AI keeps improving. ___5___ That's amazing.

Jack: That's great! Earlier detection and prediction benefit earlier treatment. It's good for all of us. ___6___

Tom: Definitely! I can't wait to see what else AI will bring to healthcare in the future.

A. It can help doctors to diagnose diseases earlier and very accurately!

B. AI can now help in surgery with amazing precision!

C. AI makes healthcare more efficient.

D. It can provide personalized treatment.

Dialogue Three

Robert: AI in medicine is becoming a hot topic recently. What amazing technology!

Andrew: Yes, people talk about it a lot. But I'm not very optimistic about its application.

Robert: Why? It could help doctors diagnose diseases better.

Andrew: ___7___ but there are a lot of potential downsides too. AI is only as good as the data it's trained on, and that data might be biased or incomplete.

Robert: But doctors could check the data first.

Andrew: ___8___ But AI doesn't have the same common sense as humans. It might make mistakes doctors wouldn't.

Robert: Sometimes people make mistakes too. What about personalized treatments?

Andrew: ___9___ but we don't really know how it would work in practice. And there are ethical concerns about using AI without patients' full informed consent.

Robert: ___10___ It seems like a double-edged sword. We need to be careful how we use AI in medicine.

Andrew: Absolutely. We can't sacrifice patient safety and privacy just to save time or money.

A. Hmm, I see your point.

B. That sounds good in theory.

C. Sure, they could,

D. That's true.

Reading & Writing

Text A

Artificial Intelligence in Healthcare

In recent years, artificial intelligence (AI) has grown rapidly and has been widely used in many fields. It has especially <u>captured the public's attention</u> in healthcare. Within the healthcare industry, AI is used in four distinct categories: living assistance, biomedical information processing, research activities, and diagnosis and prediction of diseases.

Living assistance: AI is <u>playing a</u> crucial <u>role in</u> enhancing the quality of life for the elderly and individuals with disabilities. For instance, a fall-detection system uses a software called "radar Doppler" to reduce fall risks among the elderly. <u>With the help of</u> "ambient intelligent systems" , visually impaired individuals can integrate seamlessly into communities with fully sighted individuals, even in specific professional domains. Additionally, human-machine interfaces now have the ability to interpret <u>facial expressions</u> and <u>translate</u> them <u>into</u> commands, allowing individuals with disabilities to operate their wheelchairs independently, without <u>relying on</u> sensors.

Biomedical information processing: <u>When it comes to</u> biomedical question answering, being accurate and fast is crucial for addressing different user inquiries. This can be a challenging task, but advancements in natural language processing have made it easier. First, we gather biomedical information from various sources to create a comprehensive document database. This <u>used to</u> be a time-consuming process of comparing, merging, and filtering documents. But now, with the help of artificial intelligence, we can do it much more quickly and precisely. Next, machine learning algorithms help us <u>group</u> biomedical questions <u>into</u> categories. Then, a smart system jumps in to find the right documents for each question. It quickly searches through the questions and <u>matches</u> them <u>with</u> the right documents to find the information needed for an answer. By combining these technologies, we can ensure that users get quick and accurate answers to their biomedical questions.

Research activities: AI is a very helpful tool in biomedic research. It can help researchers quickly screen, index, and rank <u>academic literature</u>. With AI's help, researchers can formulate hypotheses faster and test them more thoroughly. Modern medical devices are becoming "smarter", which helps researchers create <u>simulation models,</u> speeding up the whole research process. Additionally, AI-powered machines make it easier for researchers to understand complex information in fields like biomedical imaging, oral surgery, and <u>plastic surgery</u> by providing intuitive images.

Diagnosis and prediction of diseases: The most amazing application of AI in healthcare is its ability to diagnose diseases. AI has already made a lot of amazing breakthroughs in this area. It can help doctors diagnose many diseases earlier and more accurately. For example, AI can analyze <u>gene expression</u> data to find out if a person has cancer or not. It can even predict how long a cancer patient will live. Plus, with the help of AI and biosensors, doctors can now detect heart disease earlier than ever before.

AI plays a crucial role in diagnosing diseases through medical imaging. It excels in processing biomedical images with high accuracy, efficiency, and reliability. For example, Mayo Clinic has developed an AI system that can identify precancerous changes in a woman's cervix. This system has a higher success rate than human experts, achieving 91% accuracy compared to the human expert's 69%. Epilepsy, a condition characterized by unpredictable and recurrent seizures, has been a challenging condition to treat. However, with the help of intracranial electroencephalography (iEEG) recordings and AI techniques, it is now possible to predict the possibility of seizure.

AI in healthcare has enormous potential and is only growing stronger. The future of healthcare is bound to be interconnected with AI.

(577 words)

New Words

artificial [ˌɑːtɪˈfɪʃl]	**adj.**人造的；不自然的
intelligence [ɪnˈtelɪdʒəns]	**n.**聪颖；智力；情报
industry [ˈɪndəstri]	**n.**工业；产业
distinct [dɪˈstɪŋkt]	**adj.**不同的；清楚的，明显的；确切的
category [ˈkætəgəri]	**n.**种类；类别
assistance [əˈsɪstəns]	**n.**帮助；援助；支持；资助
biomedical [ˌbaɪəʊˈmedɪkl]	**adj.**（有关）生物医学的
processing [ˈprəʊsesɪŋ]	**n.**（数据）处理；整理；配置；工艺（生产方法）设计
process [ˈprəʊses , prəˈses]	**n.**过程；变化过程；做事方法
	v.加工；处理；冲印；审核；列队行进
diagnosis [ˌdaɪəgˈnəʊsɪs]	**n.**诊断；判断
diagnose [ˈdaɪəgnəʊz]	**v.** 诊断；判断
prediction [prɪˈdɪkʃn]	**n.**预报；预言；预言的事物
	v. predict [prɪˈdɪkt]　预言；预测
	adj. unpredictable [ˌʌnprɪˈdɪktəbl] 无法预言的；不可预测的
crucial [ˈkruːʃl]	**adj.**至关重要的，关键性的
enhance [ɪnˈhɑːns]	**v.**提高，增强；改进
elderly [ˈeldəli]	**adj.**年纪较大的；老人；老式的

individual [ˌɪndɪˈvɪdʒuəl]	**adj.**单独的；个人的；独特的
	n.个人；某种类型的人
disability [ˌdɪsəˈbɪləti]	**n.**缺陷；残疾；无能力；残障福利金
detection [dɪˈtekʃn]	**n.**察觉；侦破；探测；发现
	v. detect [dɪˈtekt]发现；查明；测出
Doppler [ˈdɒplə]	**adj.**（奥地利物理学家）多普勒的
ambient [ˈæmbiənt]	**adj.**周围的，包围着的；产生轻松氛围的；环境
impaired [ɪmˈpeəd]	**adj.**受损的；出毛病的；有（身体或智力）缺陷的
integrate [ˈɪntɪɡreɪt]	**v.**合并；成为一体；加入；融入群体
seamlessly [ˈsiːmləsli]	**adv.**无空隙地；无停顿地
community [kəˈmjuːnəti]	**n.**社会（团体）；共有；（生物）群落
domain [dəˈmeɪn]	**n.**领域，范围，范畴；领土
additionally [əˈdɪʃənəlɪ]	**adv.**此外
interface [ˈɪntəfeɪs]	**n.** 界面；　<计>接口；交界面
interpret [ɪnˈtɜːprət]	**v.** 诠释；领会，把…理解为；口译；演绎
command [kəˈmɑːnd]	**n.** 命令；控制；指挥部；精通
	v. 命令；赢得；控制，指挥；俯瞰
independently [ˌɪndɪˈpendəntlɪ]	**adv.**独立地，自立地，无关地
sensor [ˈsensə(r)]	**n.**传感器，灵敏元件
biosensor [biːəʊˈsensər]	**n** 生物传感器
accurate [ˈækjərət]	**adj.** 正确的，精确的；精准的
	adv. accurately [ˈækjərətlɪ] 正确无误地，准确地；精确地；如实
	n. accuracy [ˈækjərəsi] 精确（性），准确（性）；准确无误
address [əˈdres]	**n.** 地址，位置；网址；演说
	v. 写（收信人）姓名地址；解决，处理；演讲；向…说话；称呼
inquiry [ɪnˈkwaɪəri]	**n.** 调查，审查；询问，质问，质询，追究；探究；打听
challenge [ˈtʃælɪndʒ]	**n.** 挑战；比赛邀请；质疑
	v. 对…怀疑；挑战，考验；盘问
advancement [ədˈvɑːnsmənt]	**n.** 发展，推动；提升，晋升
comprehensive [ˌkɒmprɪˈhensɪv]	**adj.** 全面的；综合性的
time-consuming [ˈtaɪm kənsjuːmɪŋ]	**adj.** 费时的；旷日持久的；花费大量时间的
merge [mɜːdʒ]	**v.**（使）混合；相融；融入；渐渐消失在某物中

filter [ˈfɪltə(r)]	**n.**过滤器；筛选（过滤）程序；分流信号/指示灯
	v.过滤；渗透；泄露；仅可左转行驶
precisely [prɪˈsaɪsli]	**adv.**精确地；恰好地；严谨地，严格地；一丝不苟地
algorithm [ˈælgərɪð(ə)m]	**n.**运算法则；演算法；计算程序
combine [kəmˈbaɪn，ˈkɒmbaɪn]	**v.**使结合，混合；融合；协力，联合；同时做；（人）兼具，兼有；（使）结合；（使）联合；（使）合并；（使）综合
screen [skriːn]	**n.**屏幕；银幕；电影；屏风；掩蔽物；纱门；围屏
	v.放映；遮挡；包庇；检查；筛选；转接
index [ˈɪndeks]	**n.**索引；＜数＞指数；指示；标志
	vt.给…编索引；把…编入索引；[经济学]按生活指数调整（工资、价格等）
formulate [ˈfɔːmjuleɪt]	**vt.**构想出，规划；确切地阐述；用公式表示
hypotheses [haɪˈpɒθəsiːz]	**n.** hypothesis 的复数形式（有少量事实依据但未被证实的）假说；假设；（凭空的）猜想；猜测
AI-powered	**adj.**AI 驱动的
complex [ˈkɒmpleks]	**adj.**复杂的；复合的
	n.综合建筑群；相关联的一组事物；复合体；情结；忧虑
imaging [ˈɪmɪdʒɪŋ]	**n.**成像，镜像，映像；透视显像；意象疗法
image [ˈɪmɪdʒ]	**n.**形象；声誉；画像；雕像；塑像；映像；意象
intuitive [ɪnˈtjuːɪtɪv]	**adj.**直觉的；凭直觉获知的；直观的
amaze [əˈmeɪz]	**v.**使惊奇/惊愕
application [ˌæplɪˈkeɪʃn]	**n.**申请；请求；申请书；运用；生效
breakthrough [ˈbreɪkθruː]	**n.**重大进展；突破
analyze [ˈænəlaɪz]	**v.**分析；分解；化验
excel [ɪkˈsel]	**v.**擅长，突出；胜过
reliability [rɪˌlaɪəˈbɪlɪti]	**n.**可靠，可信赖
identify [aɪˈdentɪfaɪ]	**vt.**识别，认出；确定；使参与；把…看成一样
	vi.确定；认同
precancerous [ˌpriːˈkænsərəs]	**adj.**癌症前期的
cervix [ˈsɜːvɪks]	**n.**子宫颈；颈部
epilepsy [ˈepɪlepsi]	**n.** [医]癫痫，羊癫疯
characterize [ˈkærəktəraɪz]	**v.**使具有特点；是…的特征；描绘

recurrent [rɪˈkʌrənt]	**adj.**复发的，复现的；周期性的，经常发生的；回归的；循环的
seizure [ˈsiːʒə(r)]	**n.**没收；夺取；捕捉；突然发作
enormous [ɪˈnɔːməs]	**adj.**巨大的；极大的
interconnect [ˌɪntəkəˈnekt]	**v.**互相连接，互相联系

Phrases & Expressions

capture one's attention	引起注意
play a role in	在…中起作用
with the help of	在…的帮助下
facial expressions	面部表情
translate into	（把…）翻译成…；把…转化成
rely on	依靠，依赖
when it comes to	当提到…
used to	过去经常，曾经
group into	（使）分成；
match with	（使）与…相配，使与…较量，与…一致
academic literature	学术文献
simulation models	仿真模型
plastic surgery	整形手术
gene expression	基因表达[表现]；
compared to	与…相比，跟…相比
intracranial electroencephalography (iEEG)	颅内脑电图 (intracranial [ˌɪntrəˈkreɪnɪəl] 头颅内的，颅骨内的；electroencephalography [ɪˈlektrəʊensefəˈlɒɡrəfɪ] 脑电图学，脑电描记法；)
be bound to	很有可能，肯定会

Reading Comprehension

Choose the best answer to each of the following questions.

 1. According to the passage, what is the role of human-machine interfaces? _____

 A. They help in reducing human errors.

 B. They allow seamless integration of AI into daily life.

 C. They are not yet fully developed.

 D. They are used only for fall detection.

2.What is NOT mentioned as a benefit of using AI in biomedical information processing? _____

A. Faster processing speed.

B. Improved accuracy.

C. Better user interface design.

D. Easier grouping of questions.

3. What are the benefits of AI in biomedic research according to the passage? _____

A. It can quickly screen, index, and rank academic literature.

B. It can help doctors diagnose many diseases earlier and more accurately.

C. It creates comprehensive document databases.

D. It finds relevant documents for each question.

4. Why is AI particularly helpful in diagnosing diseases through medical imaging? _____

A. It has high accuracy, efficiency, and reliability.

B. It can process large amounts of data quickly.

C. It is interconnected with other technologies.

D. It has the ability to simulate diseases.

5. Which of the following is NOT a category where AI is used in healthcare? _____

A. Monitoring patient vital signs

B. Detecting diseases through images

C. Helping researchers test hypotheses

D. Creating social media content

Text B

AI Risks and Challenges in Clinical Setting

Artificial intelligence (AI) has many uses in healthcare, like helping with diagnosis, scientific research, drug development, medical training, and even patient self-assessment. However, the World Health Organization (WHO) warns that significant risks accompany these potential benefits.

One such risk is the inaccessibility of relevant data. AI works best with a lot of data. Ideally, AI-based systems would continuously improve as more data is added to their training sets. In reality, patient records are private, so hospitals and other institutions are reluctant to share them, and data privacy regulations restrict the availability of data in certain ways.

Another challenge lies in the quality of data used to develop algorithms. Medical records are often disorganized and might contain mistakes. Therefore, when AI systems use these data to learn, they might produce potentially distorted outcomes. Besides, if the data is collected in a biased way, the AI systems will also be biased.

Furthermore, deep learning algorithms often fail to provide convincing explanations for their predictions. Even though they make accurate predictions, it's often really hard to understand how they make those predictions. This makes it tough for doctors to fully trust AI-based decisions, especially when it comes to making important decisions. Additionally, some poor designs <u>result in</u> biased software, widening the disparities related to racial, gender and age biases in society.

Ethical concerns have been raised since AI in healthcare was first introduced. The current system requires accountability for poor decisions, especially in the medical field. However, it's not clear who should be blamed <u>in case of</u> a system failure. It might be hard to blame the doctor when they <u>had no part in</u> developing or overseeing the algorithm. <u>On the other hand</u>, faulty developers <u>seem unrelated to</u> the clinical setting. The absence of ethical guidelines for the improper use of AI in healthcare only makes things worse.

Some individuals are skeptical and even hostile to AI-based projects because they fear being replaced. The public might become disillusioned with AI if its current capabilities are overstated. Additionally, it is possible that the development and deployment of AI will be monopolized by large technology companies <u>due to</u> the financial costs of training and maintaining the models. These models, <u>regardless of</u> their benefits, might increase their power and dominance over governments and healthcare systems. The WHO also raises issues about equal <u>access to</u> these models, which could be limited by the <u>digital divide</u> and high subscription fees, making existing health disparities between developed and developing countries even worse.

Limited information exists on how AI impacts patients' final outcomes. <u>So far</u>, the majority of healthcare AI research has been conducted outside of clinical settings. Randomized controlled studies, the gold standard in medicine, can't fully demonstrate the benefits of AI in healthcare.

There are several obstacles to successfully implementing AI in the clinical sector, including data issues, developer challenges, ethical concerns, and social implications. It's important to view the adoption of AI systems in healthcare as a dynamic learning experience <u>at all levels</u>, <u>calling for</u> a more sophisticated system thinking approach in the health sector to overcome these challenges.

（511 words）

New Words

assessment [ə'sesmənt]	**n.**看法；评估；鉴定；评定；核定的付款额；估价
significant [sɪg'nɪfɪkənt]	**adj.**重要的；显著的；意味深长的
accompany [ə'kʌmpəni]	**v.**陪同，陪伴；伴随；为⋯伴奏
potential [pə'tenʃl]	**adj.**潜在的
	n.潜力；可能性
	adv. potentially [pə'tenʃəli] 潜在地；可能地
benefit ['benɪfɪt]	**n.**好处；优势；福利费；保险金；慈善活动
	v.获益
inaccessibility [ˌɪnækˌsesə'bɪlətɪ]	**n.**不易接近，难达到
relevant ['reləvənt]	**adj.**相关的；合适的；有意义
continuously [kən'tɪnjʊəsli]	**adv.**连续不断地，接连地；时时刻刻；连着
private ['praɪvət]	**adj.**私用的；私营的；个人的；秘密的；私人的；隐私的；僻静的；内敛的；间接收入的
	n. privacy ['prɪvəsi] 隐私，秘密；隐居；私事；不受公众干扰的状态
institution [ˌɪnstɪ'tjuːʃn]	**n.**机构；社会收容机构；习俗；建立；开创；制定；设立；出名的人；制度
regulation [ˌreɡju'leɪʃn]	**n.**管理；控制；规章；规则
restrict [rɪ'strɪkt]	**vt.**限制，限定；约束，束缚
availability [əˌveɪlə'bɪləti]	**n.**可用性；有效性；可得到的东西
challenge ['tʃælɪndʒ]	**n.**挑战；比赛邀请；质疑
	v.对⋯怀疑；挑战，考验；盘问
distort [dɪ'stɔːt]	**v.**歪曲，曲解；（使）变形，失真
bias ['baɪəs]	**n.**偏见；偏好
	v.使偏向
convince [kən'vɪns]	**v.**使相信；说服
disparity [dɪ'spærəti]	**n.**不同；不等；不一致；悬殊
ethical ['eθɪkl]	**adj.**伦理学的；道德的，伦理的；凭处方出售的
concern [kən'sɜːn]	**n.**担心；令人担心的事；关心（的事）；分内之事；公司
	v.影响；涉及；使担忧；关心；对⋯感兴趣；认为⋯重要

accountability [əˌkaʊntəˈbɪləti]	n.有责任，有义务；〈财〉会计责任
blame [bleɪm]	v.责怪，指责
	n.责备；（对坏事应负的）责任
oversee [ˌəʊvəˈsiː]	vt.监督，监视；俯瞰；错过，宽恕，省略
faulty [ˈfɔːlti]	adj.出故障的；有错误的
setting [ˈsetɪŋ]	n.环境；情节背景；调节点；乐曲；底座；一套餐具
absence [ˈæbsəns]	n.缺席，不在；缺乏，不存在
skeptical [ˈskeptɪkl]	adj.怀疑性的，好怀疑的，<口>无神论的
hostile [ˈhɒstaɪl]	adj.敌人的，敌对的；怀有敌意的；不利的
replace [rɪˈpleɪs]	v.替换；以…取代；更新；把…放回（原处）
disillusion [ˌdɪsɪˈluːʒn]	vt.使不再抱幻想，使理想破灭；给…泼冷水；使醒悟
overstate [ˌəʊvəˈsteɪt]	vt.夸大（某事）；把…讲得过分；夸张
deployment [dɪˈplɔɪmənt]	n.部署，调集；有效利用
monopolize [məˈnɒpəlaɪz]	vt.独占，垄断；拥有…的专卖权
financial [faɪˈnænʃl]	adj.财政的，财务的；金融的；有钱的
maintain [meɪnˈteɪn]	v.维持，保持；坚称；维修，保养；供养
dominance [ˈdɒmɪnəns]	n.支配，控制
divide [dɪˈvaɪd]	v.（使）分开；分配；除以；分隔；（使）产生分歧
	n.明显差异；分界线，分水
subscription [səbˈskrɪpʃn]	n.（报刊等的）订阅费，订阅，订购；捐款；（俱乐部的）会员费；捐助
limit [ˈlɪmɪt]	n.极限；限制；界限；范围
	v.限制；限量；使限于
impact [ˈɪmpækt , ɪmˈpækt]	n.影响；作用；冲击力
	v.对…有影响；冲击；撞击
majority [məˈdʒɒrəti]	n.多数；多数票；超出其余各方票数总和的票数
	adj.多数人支持的
conduct [kənˈdʌkt]	v.进行，组织，实施；表现，举止；指挥；传导（热或电）
randomize [ˈrændəmaɪz]	v.使随机化，完全打乱，（使）作任意排列
obstacle [ˈɒbstəkl]	n.障碍（物）；障碍物（绊脚石，障碍栅栏）
implement [ˈɪmplɪment , ˈɪmplɪmənt]	vt.实施，执行；使生效，实现；落实（政策）；把…填满
	n.工具，器械；家具；手段；[法]履行（契约等）
implication [ˌɪmplɪˈkeɪʃn]	n.含义；可能的影响（或作用、结果）；暗指；（被）牵连；[逻辑学]蕴涵，蕴含

adoption [ə'dɒpʃn]	**n.**收养，领养；采用；（候选人）选定
dynamic [daɪ'næmɪk]	**adj.**精力充沛的；活跃的；动力的；动态的
	n.动力；相互作用；驱动力；力学；力度
sophisticated [sə'fɪstɪkeɪtɪd]	**adj.**复杂的；精致的；富有经验的；深奥微妙的
overcome [ˌəʊvə'kʌm]	**v.**克服；战胜；受到…的极大影响；被熏倒

Phrases & Expressions

add to	增加，加强
in reality	实际上，事实上；实则
be reluctant to	不愿意，不情愿
in…ways	在…方式；以…方式
lie in	在于；位于；躺在；分娩
in case of	万一，如果；防备
have (no) part in	（没有）参与其中
on the other hand	在另一方面
seem/be unrelated to	似乎与…不相关
regardless of	不管；不顾
access to	接近；去…的通路，通向…的入口；有权使用，使用…的机会（权利）
digital divide	数字鸿沟
so far	到目前为止，迄今为止
at all levels	各个级别
call for	去接（某人）；去取（某物）；需要；要求

Reading Comprehension

Choose the best answer to each of the following questions.

1. The significant risks that accompany AI's potential benefits in healthcare mainly include _____.

   A. data accessibility and quality

   B. system failures and ethical concerns

   C. data privacy and biased software

   D. AI's accuracy and doctor's workload

2. According to the passage, hospitals and other institutions are reluctant to share patient records with AI-based systems mainly because _____.

A. they are not sure if AI-based systems can handle patient records well

B. they are not satisfied with AI-based systems

C. they think it is unnecessary to share data with AI-based systems

D. they want to protect patient privacy

3. The public might lose faith in AI if its current capabilities are _____.

A. misrepresented

B. underestimated

C. overestimated

D. accurately described

4. Which of the following statements is NOT true about AI development and deployment?
_____

A. It can be monopolized by large technology companies due to financial costs.

B. Models trained and maintained by AI can increase their power and dominance.

C. Equal access to AI models can be limited by digital divides and subscription fees.

D. The WHO has raised issues about equal access to AI models, making health disparities worse.

5. The author's attitude towards AI in healthcare is _____.

A. optimistic　　　　B. cautious　　　　C. critical　　　　D. subjective

Language Practice

I. Vocabulary and Structure

Directions: *Choose the one that best completes the sentence.*

1. Organic food is the food produced without _____ chemicals or pesticides.

A. human　　　　B. man　　　　C. artificial　　　　D. unreal

2. The company has successfully _____ its operations across multiple countries.

B. connected　　　　B. separated　　　　C. integrated　　　　D. divided

3. The _____ of the dolphin is very advanced, as they can communicate using sound waves.

B. language　　　　B. intelligence　　　　C. behavior　　　　D. body

4. The symptoms suggest that the patient may have a serious illness, but we can only _____ after further tests.

B. treat　　　　B. operate　　　　C. research　　　　D. diagnose

5. The presentation was so engaging that it _____ the audience's attention throughout.

B. fixed　　　　B. captured　　　　C. gained　　　　D. retained

6. AI has the potential to revolutionize healthcare, but it also raises serious _____

concerns.

    B. privacy   B. private   C. individual   D. patient

    7. The company has strict _____ on the use of social media during work hours.

    B. policies   B. measures   C. guidelines   D. regulations

    8. The reviewer's comments on the book were _____, as they did not reflect the actual content accurately.

    B. distorted   B. distinguished   C. disguised   D. distracted

    9. The new service will be launched in areas where there is good _____ of internet connectivity.

    B. prepare   B. readiness   C. suitability   D. availability

    10. All students should have equal _____ to education, regardless of their background.

    A. ability   B. access   C. capable   D. path

    11. The _____ of the company's products is increasing rapidly.

    A. request   B. demand   C. want   D. require

    12. I don't know what _____ said, but I think he was rude to the waiter.

    A. him   B. his   C. he   D. himself

    13. The _____ of the mountain range is over 2000 meters above sea level.

    A. peak height   B. high peak   C. higher peak   D. highest peak

    14. She spoke very _____ and everyone could hear her clearly.

    A. loud   B. aloud   C. loudly   D. noisy

    15. He _____ the answer to the question, but he couldn't remember it now.

    A. had known   B. has known   C. knew   D. will know

    16. The book _____ by the end of this year.

    A. is published   B. will publish

    C. has been published   D. will be published

    17. I saw him _____ the letter and put it in the envelope.

    A. write   B. writing   C. to write   D. wrote

    18. The man _____ was standing near the door is a police officer.

    A. who you saw   B. you saw him

    C. which you saw   D. that you saw him

    19. They would _____ the problem if they had more time.

    A. solve   B. have solved   C. solved   D. solving

    20. The teacher recommended that the students _____ the book before writing the report.

A. read	B. to read	C. reading	D. having read

II. Cloze

Directions: *Choose the best one to complete the passage.*

ChatGPT has many uses in healthcare, and it will probably change our healthcare systems a lot.

Doctors still need to make _____1_____ decisions about healthcare, but ChatGPT can help with clinical decisions by giving real-time, evidence-based advice. This can _____2_____ things like warning about possible drug interactions, _____3_____ different treatment options for certain conditions, and showing useful medical guidelines.

ChatGPT can also help with keeping medical records. It can sum up patients' medical history easily. Healthcare professionals can talk to ChatGPT, and it can catch important details _____4_____.

ChatGPT's ability to translate in real-time is also useful in healthcare. It can quickly and accurately translate technical terms and medical jargons _____5_____ patients will fully understand their diagnosis, treatment options, and medical instructions.

Clinical trials are important for making progress in healthcare. They help professionals find new treatments, better _____6_____ tools, and ways to prevent diseases. Finding people to take part in clinical trials can be hard, but ChatGPT could help to find patients who _____7_____ the trial criteria, making it easier for researchers to find people who want to take part.

There are online tools that help people check their symptoms and know when to seek medical attention. ChatGPT can create more accurate and reliable symptom checkers that give people _____8_____ advice about _____9_____ to do next.

ChatGPT can also help with medical education. It provides healthcare professionals and students with quick access _____10_____ important medical information and resources that support their learning and development.

1. A. final	B. end	C. last	D. decided
2. A. be included	B. include	C. including	D. includes
3. A. suggest	B. to suggest	C. suggesting	D. suggested
4. A. automation	B. automatic	C. automatical	D. automatically
5. A. so that	B. such that	C. in order that	D. for
6. A. diagnose	B. diagnosis	C. diagnoses	D. diagnostic
7. A. reach	B. equal	C. meet	D. fulfill
8. A. clear	B. clearer	C. more clear	D. most clear
9. A. when	B. what	C. where	D. how
10. A. to	B. at	C. in	D. on

III. Translation

Directions: *Translate the following passage into Chinese.*

AI is sometimes known to provide incorrect information. Dr. Taylor once asked a chat-bot to create a scientific paper summarizing opioid use disorder and to provide references. The chat-bot provided a nice summary with mostly correct information, but the references were fake. Although it listed scientist names and titles associated with existing journals, a closer inspection using search engines revealed they were invented. There are other potential source issues, too. Some users report that AI provides correct information, but the cited sources don't include the answers they asked for. Other times, users say AI provides nonexistent source links or "page not found" results. All of these make the accuracy of the answer questionable.

chatbot	聊天机器人
scientific paper	科学论文
opioid use disorder [ˈəupiɔid juːz disˈɔːdə]	**n.**阿片类物质使用障碍
reference [ˈrefrəns]	**n.**参考书目
associated with	与…有关
inspection [ɪnˈspekʃn]	**n.**检查；检验；视察；检阅
search engines	**n.**（互联网上的）搜寻引擎
invent [ɪnˈvent]	**v.**发明；编造
reveal [rɪˈviːl]	**v.**揭示；展示
cite [saɪt]	**v.**引用；引证
nonexistent [ˌnɒnɪgˈzɪstənt]	**adj.**不存在的

IV. Writing

Directions: *You are to write on the topic* **"My View on Online Chat"**. *You should base your composition on the Chinese outline given below and your essay should not be less than 100 words.*

1. 网络聊天的好处。
2. 网络聊天的坏处。
3. 我的观点。

Grammar Focus

★虚拟语气

虚拟语气用于表示与事实不相符的假设或者说话者的主观愿望。

一、与事实不相符的假设

假设是一种非真实条件，表示"如果…"，可以是对当前情况的假设、可以是对过去情况的假设，还可以是对未来情况的假设。假设条件下的结果"那么…"往往也是非真实存在的。

1. 标准假设：指假设的结果与条件在时间上同步，即对当前的假设产生当前的结果。这时英语通过谓语动词的形式变化来体现。

	假设条件（如果…）—从句	假设结果（那么…）—主句
与当前情况不相符	If+主语+动词过去式+…+,	主语+would/should/might/could+动词原形+…+.
与过去情况不相符	If+主语+had+动词过去分词+…+,	主语+would/should/might/could+ have+动词过去分词+…+.
与将来情况不相符	If+主语+were to/should+动词原形+…+，或者If+主语+动词过去式+…+,	主语+would/should/might/could+动词原形+…+.

注意：虚拟条件从句中 be 动词的过去时只有 were，没有人称和数的变化。

would（一定）/should（应该）/might（或许）/could（能够）根据句意和语气来选择，常用的是 would。

举例：If there <u>were</u> no air or water, there <u>would be</u> no living things on the earth.

如果没有空气或者水，（那么）地球上就不会有生物。（与当前情况不相符）

If I <u>had got up</u> earlier, I <u>would/might not have been</u> late for work.

如果我早点起床，（那么我）上班就不会迟到了。（与过去情况不相符，事实是我起床晚了，我已经迟到了。）

If there <u>were to be /should be /were</u> a heavy snow tomorrow, we <u>would/might make</u> a snowman on the playground.

如果明天下大雪，（那么）我们就有可能在操场上堆个雪人。（与将来情况不相符，明天下大雪的可能性很小，我们其实不可能堆雪人。）

2. 混合虚拟：指假设的条件与结果时间上不同步，此时条件从句和主句根据各自动作发生的时间分别采用上表对应的英文表达形式。

举例：

If I <u>had learned</u> medicine in my university, I <u>would be</u> a doctor now.

如果我当年在大学学医的话，（那么）我现在就是一名医生了。（条件假设与过去事实相反，结果与现在事实相反。）

If I <u>were</u> you, I <u>would have taken</u> action long ago.

如果我是你，我早就采取行动了。（条件假设与现在事实相反，结果与过去事实相反。）

3. 虚拟条件的多种表达法：

虚拟假设条件可以用 if （如果…）引导，也可以省略 if，此时从句要将 were、should、had 提前置于句首，作部分倒装处理。

例如：

Were my mother here, she would support me. (=If my mother were here, …)

我妈妈在这里的话，她会支持我的。

Had it not rained, we would have arrived on time. (=If it had not rained, …)

要是不雨的话，我们早就准时到了。

Should it be necessary, I would go to talk with him. (=If it should be necessary, …)

如果有必要，我去跟他谈谈。

If 从句也可以用暗含条件意味的短语或上下文代替，如 without（如果没有）…, but for（要不是因为）…，if only（要是…就好了），as if（仿佛，好像）等。

举例：

If there were no air or water, there would be no living things on the earth.

=Without air or water, there would be no living things on the earth.

But for your help, I would not have made such progress. (=If there were not your help, …)

要是没有你的帮助，我不会取得这样的进步。

I didn't know you were here last week, otherwise I would have invited you to dinner. (=If I had known that you were here last week, I would have invited you to dinner.)

我不知道你上周在这里，否则我会邀你一起吃饭的。

If only I had listened to my parents!

要是我当时听我父母的就好了！

She treated me as if I were a stranger.

她待我如同陌生人一般。

I'd rather I hadn't said that.

我（宁愿）真希望我没有说过那话。

二、表达说话者强烈的主观愿望

这里的主观愿望可以是主观想法、猜测或者建议等，表达主观愿望内容的谓语用 should+动词原形，有时 should 可以省略。

1. 用在宾语从句中

这类主句谓语动词常用的有 insist、order、command、advise、suggest、propose、recommend、ask、demand、require、request、move、urge、arrange、desire、intend、direct 等。

例如：

I <u>insisted</u> that I <u>(should) go</u> with them.

我坚持要同他们一起去。

The general <u>ordered</u> that the soldier <u>(should) respond</u> loudly.

将军命令士兵大声回答。

The doctor <u>advised</u> that the patient <u>(should) stop</u> smoking.

医生建议病人戒烟。

*注意：wish 引导的宾语从句按 if 条件句变化。

例如：

I <u>wish/wished</u> that the prices <u>would come</u> down.

我希望物价下降。（与现实情况相反。）

I <u>wish/wished</u> that he <u>had told</u> me the truth.

我希望他跟我讲了实话。（与过去事实相反。）

2. 用在目的状语中

引导这类目的状语的连词常用的有 for fear that、in case、lest、so that、in order that 等。

例如：

He turned his phone to silent mode <u>lest</u> the ringtone <u>(should) disturb</u> the meeting.

他把手机调为静音，以免会议被铃声干扰。

The teacher explained that passage again and again <u>in order that</u> every student <u>(might) understand</u> it.

为了让每位学生都听懂，老师反反复复地讲那一段。

3. 用在定语从句中：

常用句型是 It is/was (high) time that…表示该是…的时间了。

例如：

It's already twelve hours at night. <u>It's high time that</u> you <u>(should) go</u> to bed.

已是夜里十二点了，该是上床睡觉的时间了。

4. 用在主语从句中：

常用句型是 It is … that +主语从句，be 联系动词后面往往是表示情绪或观点的形容词或者动词。

例如：

It is <u>the best</u> that we <u>(should) make</u> a decision right now.

最好我们立刻做决定。

It was <u>proposed</u> that the meeting <u>(should) be</u> postponed.

有人提议将会议延期。

It is <u>a pity</u> that he <u>(should) fail</u> the exam.

他考试没及格，真遗憾。

Have a check on your grammar 过关演练

Directions: *Choose the best answer to complete the sentence.*

1. If he _____ the answer, he would have raised his hand.

A. know　　　B. knows　　　C. knew　　　D. had known

2. If he _____ ill, he would have come to the party.

A. isn't　　　B. wasn't　　　C. weren't　　　D. hasn't been

3. If I had enough money, I _____ that car.

A. buy　　　B. will buy　　　C. would buy　　　D. would have bought

4. If _____ you, I would go on holiday to Hainan.

A. I were　　　B. Were I　　　C. I am　　　D. Am I

5. She speaks English as if she _____ a native speaker.

A. were　　　B. was　　　C. is　　　D. had been

6. The doctor suggested that he _____ for a walk at least half an hour every day.

A. go　　　B. goes　　　C. went　　　D. have gone

7. —Shall I open the window?

—I'd rather you _____.

A. can't　　　B. won't　　　C. didn't　　　D. hadn't

8. It's possible that he _____us some money, but it's impossible that he _____us so much.

A. will lend, will lend　　　B. will lend, should lend

C. should lend, will lend　　　D. should lend, should lend

9. Thank you very much indeed. Bur for your advice, I really _____what I should have done.

A. don't know　　　B. didn't know

C. hadn't known　　　D. wouldn't have known

10. Read in a good light lest it _____ your eyes.

A. hurts　　　B. will hurt　　　C. had hurt　　　D. should hurt

附 录

常用口语表达

Have a nice day. 祝你今天愉快。

How's it going? 近况如何？

So far, so good. 目前为止一切都好。

Keep it up! 继续努力，继续加油！

Time flies! 时光如梭，时光飞逝。

Time is money. 时间就是金钱。

The best things in life are free. 生命中最好的东西是金钱买不到的。

Let's go with the flow. 让一切顺其自然吧。

That's life. 这就是人生。

I'm so proud of you. 我为你感到骄傲。

The rest is history. 众所皆知。

Hang in there. 坚持下去。

It never rains but it pours. 祸不单行。

It's a long story. 说来话长。

Are you free tonight? 你今晚有空吗？

How was your day? 你今天过得怎么样？

It was nice talking to you. 和你聊天很愉快。

What's your plan for the weekend? 你周末有什么计划？

What are you going to do next? 你接下来要做什么？

How do you usually spend your weekend? 你平时周末都怎么度过？

It slipped my mind. 我忘了。

You can't please everyone. 你不可能讨好每一个人。

I'll keep my ears open. 我会留意的。

What a small world! 世界真小！

Could be worse. 可能更糟。

Go fifty-fifty on something. 平分。

Can you give me a hand? 你能帮帮我吗？

You can say that again! You said it! 你说的没错!

Take my word for it. 相信我的话。

What's up? 有什么新鲜事吗?

What do you do for a living? 你做什么工作?

Sorry, I'm late. 对不起，我迟到了。

What's that? 那是什么?

I like your sense of humour. 我喜欢你的幽默感。

I'll call you. 我会打电话给你。

I would like to talk to you for a minute. 我想和你谈一下。

May I see your passport, please? 请给我你的护照?

Where are you staying? 将在哪儿住宿?

Where can I get my baggage? 我在何处可取得行李?

I'm an office worker. 我是上班族。

I work for the government. 我在政府机关做事。

I have a lot of problems. 我有很多问题。

I'm looking forward to seeing you. 我期望见到你。

I'm supposed to go on a diet / get a raise. 我应该节食/涨工资。

I see what your mean. 我了解你的意思。

I can't do this. 我不能这么做。

Let me explain why I was late. 让我解释迟到的理由。

Where is your office? 你们的办公室在哪?

Can you help me? 你能帮助我吗?

Can you repeat that? 你能重复一遍吗?

That's interesting. 那很有趣。

I can't wait. 我等不及了。

It's easier said than done. 说起来容易做起来难。

I'm all ears. 我洗耳恭听。

Better luck next time. 下次运气更好。

Come in handy. 派得上用场。

Rain cats and dogs. 倾盆大雨。

Not yet. 还没。

Allow me. 让我来。

Be quiet! 安静点!

Good job! 做得好!

Have fun! 玩得开心!

How much? 多少钱?

I'm full. 我饱了。

I'm home. 我回来了。

My treat. 我请客。

This way, please. 这边请。

After you. 您先。

Slow down! 慢点!

Try again. 再试试。

Be careful! 小心!

Bottoms up! 干杯(见底)!

Don't move! 不许动!

Guess what? 猜猜看?

Let me see. 让我想想。

I'm bored. 我很无聊。

I'm so tired. 我好累。

Let's hang out. 我们一起出去玩吧。

What's on your mind? 你在想什么?

Meet a deadline. 按期完成。

Go from bad to worse. 每况愈下。

Hit the jackpot. 中大奖,走运。

The tip of the iceberg. 冰山一角。

Behind the scenes. 在幕后。

I don't have a clue. 我一点头绪都没有。

You never know what you can do until you try. 不试试看,就不知道自己的潜力。

Can I take a rain check? 能改天吗?

Make a mountain out of a molehill. 大惊小怪;小题大做;言过其实。

Keep an eye on it. 留意一下。

Shake a leg. 快点,动起来(适合用在家人和老朋友之间)。

Two heads are better than one. 三个臭皮匠抵过一个诸葛亮。

Through thick and thin. 历尽千辛万苦。

All in the day's work. 司空见惯。

Under the weather. 不舒服。

Let's grab a bite. 我们去吃点东西吧。

It doesn't matter. 没关系。

That's awesome! 太棒了！

I'm sorry to hear that. 听到这个我很难过。

See you later. 再见。

I'm just kidding. 我只是开玩笑的。

Don't worry about it. 别担心。

I'm on my way. 我在路上。

Curiosity killed the cat. 好奇害死猫。

Great minds think alike. 英雄所见略同。

There's no place like home. 没有一个地方可以和家相提并论。

It takes two to tango. 孤掌难鸣。

Some people have all the luck. 有些人总是那么幸运。

Don't be such a poor loser. 不要输不起。

Don't cry over spilt milk. 覆水难收。

It wouldn't hurt to ask. 问也无妨。

Have one's head in the clouds. 心不在焉。

Never say die. 决不要灰心。

Seeing is believing. 眼见为实。

Patience is a virtue. 耐心是一种美德。

Talk is cheap. 光说没有用。

Turn over a new leaf. 洗心革面。

Burn the midnight oil. 挑灯夜战。

Something is better than nothing. 有总比没有强。

The calm before the storm. 暴风雨前的宁静。

The early bird catches the worm. 早起的鸟儿有虫吃。

Tomorrow is another day. 明天又是崭新的一天。

Do you have any pets? 你有宠物吗？

What's your favorite animal? 你最喜欢的动物是什么？

Where would you like to travel? 你想去哪里旅行？

Can you speak another language? 你会说其他语言吗？

What's your favorite sport? 你最喜欢的运动是什么？

What's the best restaurant in town? 这个城市最好的餐厅在哪里？

Do you have any siblings? 你有兄弟姐妹吗？

What's your favorite season? 你最喜欢的季节是什么？

Come out in the wash. 真相大白。

Every dog has his day. 人皆有得意时。

Bury the hatchet. 言归于好。

In the nick of time. 及时。

Don't speak too soon. 别说得太早。

Sell like hot cakes. 很畅销。

Look before you leap. 三思而后行。

Bet one's bottom dollar. 打包票。

A wolf in sheep's clothing. 披着羊皮的狼。

Haste makes waste. 欲速则不达。

Someone is not out of the woods yet. 还未脱离危险。

Easy come, easy go. 易得易失。

Practice makes perfect. 熟能生巧。

On the spur of the moment. 一时冲动；一时兴起。

Every little bit counts. 一点一滴都算。

That's a good idea. 那是个好主意。

In the same boat. 处境相同，面临同样的困境。

Appearances can be deceiving. 外表是会骗人的。

Don't put all your eggs in one basket. 别孤注一掷。

Take the bull by the horns. 当机立断；临危不惧。

Excuse me, is there… nearby? 请问附近有没有…？

Excuse me, how do I get to the…?　请问如何前往…？

An eye for an eye, and a tooth for a tooth. 以眼还眼，以牙还牙。

Money doesn't grow on trees. 挣钱不容易。

Not get a word in edgewise. 插不上话。

I have no idea. 我不知道。

That's incredible. 真不可思议。

It's a piece of cake. 这太容易了。

Take it easy. 别紧张。

It's none of your business. 这不关你的事。

I'm so excited! 我太兴奋了！

That's a shame. 真遗憾。

How's your family? 你家人怎么样？

I'm not feeling well. 我感觉不舒服。

What's the matter? 怎么了？

Are you serious? 你是认真的吗？

I can't believe my eyes. 我不敢相信我的眼睛。

That's the way it is. 就是这样。

What's the catch? 有什么内幕吗？

Go back to square one. 回到原地。

It's never too late to learn. 学习永远不嫌晚。

Leave well enough alone. 顺其自然，安于现状。

Nothing to write home about. 没什么好写的。

Packcd in like sardines. 挤得要命。

There are other fish in the sea. 天涯何处无芳草。

What you see is what you get. 你看到什么就是什么。

It's not the end of the world. 不是世界末日。

Come away empty-handed. 一无所获。

Breathe down someone's neck. 对某人盯紧。

Fill someone's shoes. 接替某人的职位。

Act the mustard. 达到标准。

Like a dream come true. 如梦成真。

All systems are go. 准备好了。

Just what the doctor ordered. 正合需要。

The first step is always the hardest. 万事开头难。

Time changes, people change. 时间会变，人也会变。

She turns me off. 她使我厌烦。

Be my guest. 请便，别客气。

That was a close call. 太危险了／千钧一发。

Far from it. 一点也不。

I'm broke. 我破产了。

I'm lost. 我迷路了。

I'm so done with this. 我真是受够了。

I'm in a hurry. 我很匆忙。

I'm speechless. 我无言以对。

It's a pain in the neck. 真让人头疼。

My mouth is watering！我要流口水了！

I ache all over. 我浑身酸痛。

I have a runny nose. 我流鼻涕。

Do you have any openings? 你们（职位）有空缺吗？

Think nothing of it. 别放在心上。

I'm not myself today. 我今天心神不宁。

Don't beat around the bush. 别拐弯抹角了。

It's up on the air. 尚未确定。

What's the big deal? 有什么大不了的？

I have a sweet tooth. 我爱吃甜食。

That's a good question. 这是个好问题。

Let's make a deal. 我们就这么办吧。

It's not my cup of tea. 这不是我的菜。

What's the purpose of your visit? 你来访的目的是什么？

How long are you staying? 你要在这里待多久？

What's your favorite movie? 你最喜欢的电影是什么？

What do you recommend? 你有什么推荐？

Can you speak louder, please? 你能大声一点吗？

Neck and neck. 势均力敌。

I'm feeling under the weather. 我觉得不舒服 / 精神不好 / 情绪低落。

Don't get me wrong. 不要误会我。

You're the boss. 听你的。

It'll come to me. 我会想起来的。

I'm so over it. 我对这事真是彻底无语了。

It's a long shot. 这是个不太可能成功的尝试。

Let's hit the road. 我们出发吧。

I'm on cloud nine. 我非常快乐。

It's a small world after all. 毕竟世界很小。

What a pain! 多痛苦啊！

Let's hit the hay. 我们去睡觉吧。

It's a no-brainer. 这是很容易的事。

Piece of cake! 小菜一碟！

The ball is in your court. 你现在掌握主动权。

Easy does it. 慢慢来，不着急。

Give it a shot. 试一试吧。

Hush-hush. 保密。

I will play it by ear. 我会见机行事的；到时候再说。

Let's give him a big hand. 让我们热烈鼓掌。

As far as I'm concerned. 就我而言。

Let the cat out of the bag. 泄露秘密。

Out of the blue. 出乎意料。

Pick up the slack. 补足不足之处。

The more, the merrier. 人多热闹。

Hold on. 等一等。

I agree. 我同意。

Not bad. 还不错。

Burn the midnight oil. 通宵达旦的学习。

Go the extra mile. 努力做更多。

Hit the nail on the head. 说到点子上。

In a nutshell. 简而言之。

Jump to conclusions. 草率下结论。

Do you like cooking? 你喜欢做饭吗？

I'm in. 我加入。

I'll pass. 我就不参加了。

Just to be on the safe side. 为了安全起见。

It's been a long time. 好久不见了。

It's about time. 时间差不多了。

I can't imagine why .我想不通为什么。

That's really something. 真了不起。

Excuse me for a moment. 失陪一会儿。

I see. 我明白了。

I'm dying to see you. 我真想见你。

It can't be helped. 无能为力。

I quit! 我不干了!

Sorry to bother you. 抱歉打扰你。

Stay out of this matter, please. 请别管这事。

I'll make it up to you. 我会赔偿的。

Let go! 放手!

Let's forgive and forget. 让我们摈弃前嫌。

I've heard so much about you! 久仰大名。

Don't underestimate me. 别小看我。

She gives me a headache. 她让我头疼。

Don't get on my nerves! 不要搅得我心烦。

His argument doesn't hold water. 他的论点站不住脚。

That's all! 就这样!

Time is up. 时间快到了。

What 's new? 有什么新鲜事吗?

Count me on. 算上我。

Feel better? 好点了吗?

I'm his fan. 我是他的影迷。

Make it short.长话短说吧。

Thank you for your company. 谢谢你陪我。

Maybe next time. 要不下次吧?

I won't be long. 我很快就好。

I gotta take off. 我得走了。

It's up to you. 你决定。

You suck! 你真差劲儿。

Rain check? 要不改日再约?

Shut it! / Shut up! 闭嘴。

My bad. 我的错。

Not your concern. 不关你的事儿。

No comment. 无可奉告。

Shame on you! 真为你感到羞耻。

Says who? 谁说的?

Since when? 从什么时候开始的?

Where to? 到哪儿?

Whatever you say! 你说什么就是什么!

I give you my word/ You have my word. 我向你保证。

Not even close. 差得还远着呢。

What are the odds? 这也太巧了吧!

What's in it for me? 对我有什么好处?

Feather in one's cap. 值得骄傲的成就。

It's a piece of art. 这是一件艺术品。

Jump on the bandwagon. 赶时髦。

Keep your chin up. 保持乐观。

Put your thinking cap on. 动动脑筋。

Run out of steam. 筋疲力尽。

Vanish into thin air. 消失得无影无踪。

When pigs fly. 无稽之谈。

You've hit the nail on the head. 你说到点子上了。

A picture is worth a thousand words. 百闻不如一见。

Don't count your chickens before they hatch. 不要过早乐观。

Fortune favors the bold. 天助勇者。

In the heat of the moment. 一时冲动。

Make a long story short. 长话短说。

Out of the frying pan, into the fire. 跳进火坑。

Practice what you preach. 身教胜于言传。

Rome wasn't built in a day. 伟业非一日之功。

Strike while the iron is hot. 趁热打铁。

Variety is the spice of life. 多样化是生活的调味品。

Weather the storm. 渡过难关。

A penny for your thoughts. 出个主意吧。

Back to the drawing board. 重新开始。

Get your act together. 有条不紊地行事。

I'm heading out for a bit. 我要外出一会儿。

Let's take a spontaneous road trip. 我们来一次即兴的公路之旅吧。

I'm off on a business trip next week. 我下周要出差。

I'll be on the move for the next few days. 我接下来几天会一直在外面。

I'm going on vacation to recharge. 我要度假来充电。

Excuse me, can you show me the way? 对不起，你能告诉我怎么走吗？

Can you recommend a good restaurant? 你能推荐一个好餐厅吗？

Can you give me a discount? 你能给我打个折吗？

I need some help. 我需要帮助。

I had a nightmare. 我做了个可怕的梦。

You forgot to turn off the light. 你忘关灯了。

You owe me one. 你欠我一个人情。

I don't mean it. 我不是故意的。

I'll fix you up. 我会帮你打点的。

You can make it! 你能做到!

Control yourself! 克制一下!

How's everything? 一切还好吧?

I'll try my best. 我尽力而为。

What a good deal! 真便宜!

You asked for it! 你自讨苦吃!

That's all I need. 我就要这些。

The view is great. 景色多么漂亮!

Any messages for me? 有我的留言吗?

Don't give me that! 少来这套!

It is growing cool. 天气渐渐凉爽起来。

How are things going? 事情进展得怎样?

I know all about it. 我知道有关它的一切。

It really takes time. 这样太耽误时间了。

It's against the law. 这是违法的。

Great minds think alike. 英雄所见略同。

I really enjoyed myself. 我玩得很开心。

I'm fed up with my work! 我对工作烦死了!

It's no use complaining. 发牢骚没什么用。

I'll just play it by ear. 我到时随机应变。

I'm not sure I can do it. 恐怕这事我干不了。

Let's not waste our time. 咱们别浪费时间了。

May I ask some questions? 我可以问几个问题吗?

I saw it with my own eyes. 我亲眼所见。

I will arrange everything. 我会安排一切的。

I would like to check out. 我想结账（退房）。

Show your tickets, please! 请出示你的票!

Thank you for your advice. 谢谢你的建议。

That's the latest fashion. 这是最流行的款式。

The train arrived on time. 火车准时到达。

Things are getting better. 情况正在好转。

Close-up. 特写镜头。

Any urgent thing? 有急事吗?

How about eating out? 去外面吃饭怎样?

I'm afraid I can't. 我恐怕不能。

You want a bet? 你想打赌吗?

Come seat here. 来这边坐。

I wonder if you can give me a lift? 能让我搭一程吗?

Can I have this? 可以给我这个吗?

Why are you so sure? 怎么这样肯定?

Don't get loaded. 别喝醉了。

Right over there. 就在那里。

Doggy bag. 打包袋。

Pull over! 靠边停车。

Does it serve your purpose? 对你有用吗?

You ask for it! 活该!

Thousand times no! 绝对办不到!

It is urgent. 有急事。

Say hello to everybody for me. 替我向大家问好。

Not precisely! 不见得,不一定!

He has a quick eye. 他的眼睛很锐利。

What brought you here? 什么风把你吹来了?

I'll get even with him one day. 我总有一天跟他扯平。

You don't seem to be quite yourself today. 你今天看起来不大对劲。

Do you have any money on you? 你身上带钱了吗?

I swear by the God. 我对天发誓。

You might at least apologize. 你顶多道个歉就得了。

She is still mad at me. 她还在生我的气。

Let's play it by ear. 让我们随兴所至。

Hit the ceiling. 大发雷霆。

Don't play possum! 别装蒜!

She'll be along in a few minutes. 她马上会过来。

I don't have anywhere to be. 没地方可去。

Would you mind making less noise? 能不能小声点?

Tell me when! 随时奉陪!

Better late than never. 迟做比不做好;亡羊补牢。

Don't take it out on me. 别拿我当出气筒。

Cat got your tong? 哑口无言了吧?/无话可说了吧?

Don't patronize me. 别敷衍我。

Don't put yourself down. 不必妄自菲薄。

I have a crush on you. 我对你倾心不已。

Let bygones be bygones. 过去的事就让它过去吧。

We are on the same page. 达成共识/合拍。

I get the picture. 我了解了。

I'll cut to the chase. 我就有话直说/开门见山。

We are good to go. 我们准备就绪了。

Your silence speaks volumes. 你的沉默表明了一切。

Could you scoot over? 麻烦挪一下。

What are you getting at? 你在暗示什么？

Dazzle me！ 用你的想法惊艳我吧！

You forced my hand. 你逼我的。

Let's get down to business. 我们言归正传吧。

Who would have thought? 谁能想到？

Don't make up a story. 不要捏造事实。

Do you have straw？ 你有吸管吗？

I will leave you to it. 那我就不打扰了。

You are the love of my life. 你是我的一生挚爱。

Fingers crossed. 祝你一切顺利。

A blank check. 全权处理。

Bag of tricks. 各种诀窍，种种手法。

Beat a dead horse. 徒劳无功。

To ask for the moon. 异想天开。

Strike while the iron is hot. 趁热打铁。

Ahead of the game. 处于有利地位。

Add insult to injury. 雪上加霜。

A balancing act. 权衡各种因素，兼顾各个方面。

Once in a blue moon. 千载难逢。

To take someone's word for it. 相信某人说的话。

To stick around. 就是继续在这里待下去。

Where did you grow up? 你在哪儿长大？

We all know each other pretty well. 我们彼此之间有很深的了解。

I hope our dreams come true. 我希望我梦想成真。

反侵权盗版声明

电子工业出版社依法对本作品享有专有出版权。任何未经权利人书面许可，复制、销售或通过信息网络传播本作品的行为；歪曲、篡改、剽窃本作品的行为，均违反《中华人民共和国著作权法》，其行为人应承担相应的民事责任和行政责任，构成犯罪的，将被依法追究刑事责任。

为了维护市场秩序，保护权利人的合法权益，我社将依法查处和打击侵权盗版的单位和个人。欢迎社会各界人士积极举报侵权盗版行为，本社将奖励举报有功人员，并保证举报人的信息不被泄露。

举报电话：（010）88254396；（010）88258888

传　　真：（010）88254397

E-mail：　dbqq@phei.com.cn

通信地址：北京市万寿路 173 信箱

　　　　　电子工业出版社总编办公室

邮　　编：100036